TEEN PEOPLE
Celebrity Beauty Guide

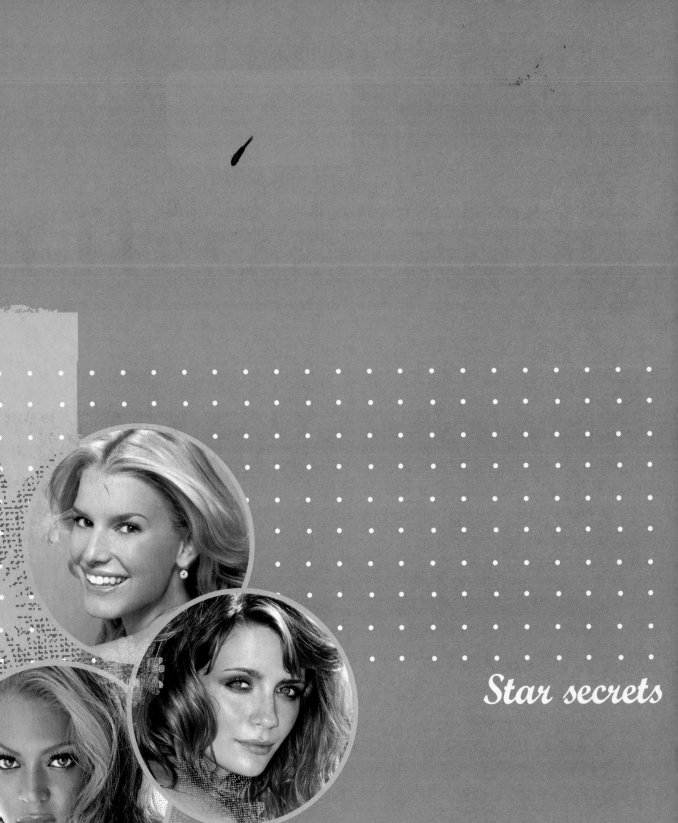

Star secrets

Teen People

CELEBRITY BEAUTY GUIDE

From the Editors of Teen People magazine
with Lauren McCann and Maria Neuman

for gorgeous hair, makeup, skin, and more!

STARRING: JESSICA SIMPSON · BEYONCÉ · LINDSAY LOHAN · MISCHA BARTON · HILARY DUFF

ASHANTI · MANDY MOORE · GWEN STEFANI · KATE BOSWORTH · PINK · SARAH MICHELLE GELLAR

LUCY LIU · AVRIL LAVIGNE · DREW BARRYMORE · JENNIFER ANISTON · EVE · KIRSTEN DUNST

JENNIFER LOPEZ · ASHLEE SIMPSON · CHRISTINA AGUILERA · JENNIFER GARNER ·

PARIS HILTON · KELLY ROWLAND · RAVEN . . .

Teen People CELEBRITY BEAUTY GUIDE

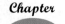
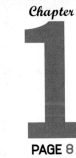
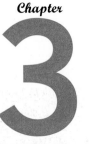

Contents

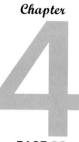
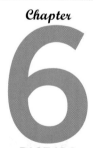
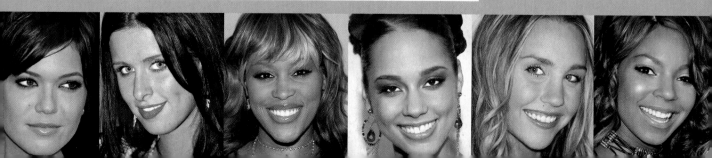

INTRO-DUCTION

Look at you!

Chances are you've got something beautiful in common with your favorite celebrity. After all, today's definition of pretty is so big—every time you flip on the TV, go to the movies, or catch a concert or video, you see yourself represented. Beauty is all skin colors, all hair types, all shapes and sizes. So maybe your eyes are the same color as the star you love, or your curls have the same texture. Or maybe, just like that fabulous celeb, you get zits . . . or split ends . . . or broken nails. Because, believe it or not, the rich and famous are not immune to these baffling beauty dilemmas!

In fact, the only difference between you and your celeb role models is that they've got a whole squad of experts who work night and day to make them red-carpet ready. Really—think about how hot you'd look if you had your own personal staff of stylists to get you gorgeous before school in the morning! **Well, this book is the next best thing.**

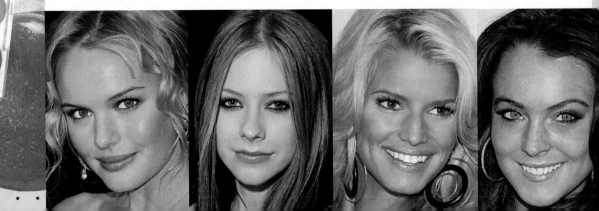

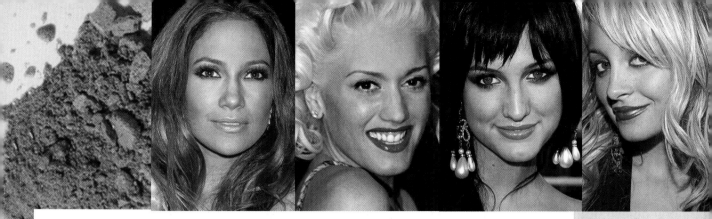

Since no one gets closer to the stars than we do at TEEN PEOPLE magazine, we decided to use our celebrity access to your advantage. We chose the most beautiful people in entertainment, met with the pros who do their hair, makeup, skin, and more—and learned all their secrets! Then we broke everything down into fun, easy how-tos you can do (and afford!) right now . . .

Plus, we packed our book with quizzes and party ideas and other cool stuff to make getting glam even more of a blast! So whether you're aiming for a total makeover or just want to look like a diva for the night, we've got all the info you need to get ready for your close-up—*every single day!*

Amy Barnett
Managing Editor

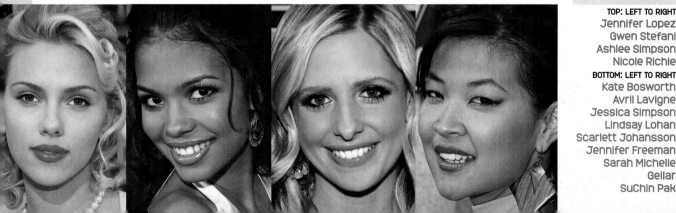

TOP: LEFT TO RIGHT
Jennifer Lopez
Gwen Stefani
Ashlee Simpson
Nicole Richie
BOTTOM: LEFT TO RIGHT
Kate Bosworth
Avril Lavigne
Jessica Simpson
Lindsay Lohan
Scarlett Johansson
Jennifer Freeman
Sarah Michelle
Gellar
Suchin Pak

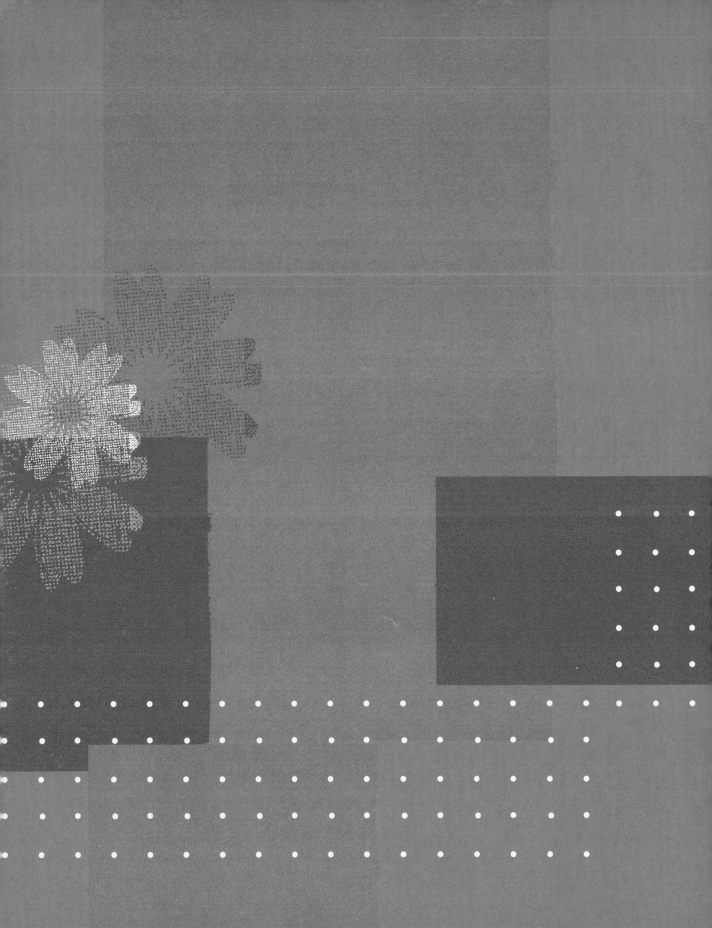

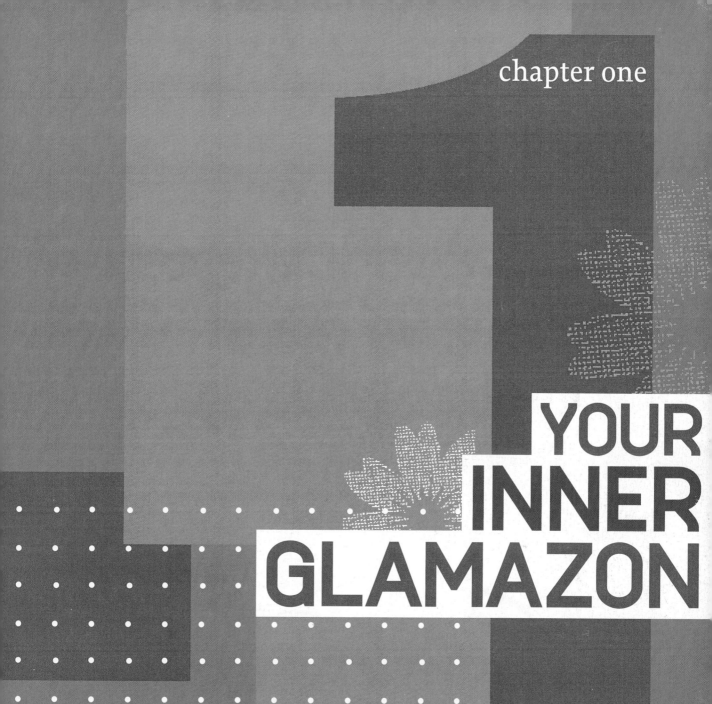

chapter one

YOUR INNER GLAMAZON

how to find, feel, and work your natural gorgeousness

OUR ALL-TIME FAVORITE GLAMOUR GIRLS

*S*ome people just have it. "It" being not one thing in particular, but lots of things that seem to make the spotlight shine a little brighter on them, like perfect hair, pearly white teeth, or mesmerizing eyes. Sometimes you can't even put your finger on "it." It's just there. It goes beyond appearance–like enormous talent, relentless drive, and that special inner something that draws you to them! Here are some glamour girls who we think really, really have "it."

Beyoncé

WHY SHE ROCKS:

- She flaunts her curves. Her body is bodacious and beautiful.

- She changes up her look. We've seen her hair go from silky straight to cutely curled in the course of an evening.

- Her voice is impossible to typecast. Beyoncé can belt out tunes with that fabulous voice of hers in tons of different genres, from hip-hop to R & B.

- She's really funny! She was hysterical as Foxy Cleopatra in *Austin Powers: Goldmember,* proving she can act as well as sing!

Jessica Simpson

WHY SHE ROCKS:

- She doesn't quit. After flopping as a kid at auditions for *The Mickey Mouse Club,* she tried again and again, not giving up until she hit the big time.

- She keeps her body in tip-top form. Jessica takes a speed walk or jog whenever she can.

- She's a writer. Not only does she entertain us on MTV's *Newlyweds,* she is about to coauthor a book with her husband on relationship advice. This will be her second book.

- She's just gorgeous. Do her hair and skin ever look bad? After watching her day in and day out on the tube, we don't think so.

Liv Tyler

WHY SHE ROCKS:

- Her skin is flawless and glowing without a drop of makeup.

- She's got amazing eyes. They are so deep blue, you can't help but stare at them.

- She's a great actress. She swept us away as the pointy-eared elf Arwen Evenstar in *The Lord of the Rings* and warmed our hearts in *Jersey Girl* (her costar, Ben Affleck, warmed our hearts too!).

- She's not afraid to take a stand. Since she is such an animal lover, she won't eat meat.

WHY SHE ROCKS:

- She has fun with her hair. It's constantly changing from blond to brown to a combination of the two, and from curly to straight.

- She's got great lips. They always look like they are puckered—even when they're not.

- She's a talented—and funny—actress. She cracked us up in *The Cookout* and *Barbershop*.

- She's tough and sweet—all at once. Her nickname is "Pit Bull in a Skirt." Need we say more?

Eve

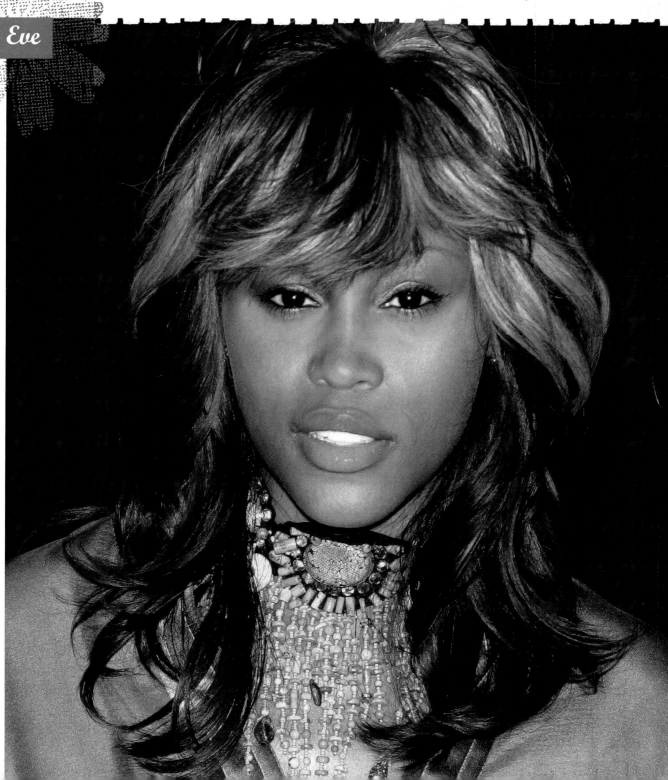

Mischa Barton

WHY SHE ROCKS:

- She's got fabulous cheekbones. They are so chiseled, Mischa never needs to use blush.

- She's got great taste. Her makeup and clothes are always understated and complement—never overpower—her assets, like a great body and huge almond eyes.

- Her hair always looks perfect! Whether it's wavy, straight, hanging down, or upswept, it always looks just right.

- She's a closet sketch artist. In her downtime, she's really into drawing people's faces.

Gwen Stefani

WHY SHE ROCKS:

- She wears bright red lipstick every day—no matter what she is doing! And she pulls it off beautifully.

- She transforms her image all the time. One day she is a rocker chick, the next, a glamour queen.

- She's got gorgeous abs. And she's not scared to show off her six-pack by wearing shirts that reveal her belly.

- She has her own cool fashion label, L.A.M.B., which makes everything from tees to tote bags.

- She's confident. She wasn't afraid to take a break from the guys in No Doubt to release a solo album.

QUIZ: WHO IS YOUR BEAUTY ROLE MODEL?

We all love looking through the pages of **Teen People** every month and spying the newest celeb-tested hair and makeup ideas. Whose looks do you love? Are you a natural wonder who loves unfussy hair and barely-there makeup, like Cameron Diaz, or a glamour girl who likes nothing better than road-testing Christina Aguilera's latest pink lips and long lashes? Take the quiz below and find out which star you most relate to when it comes to beauty, as well as discover easy ideas on how to show off your own style.

1. WHAT IS YOUR FAVORITE BEAUTY PRODUCT?
A) A good moisturizer
B) A little pot of loose glitter
C) A shimmer cream that works on cheeks and lips
D) Black eyeliner

2. WHAT DO YOU DO AFTER SCHOOL?
A) Cruise the mall with friends
B) A couple of hours of volunteer work
C) Burn CDs at home
D) My nails

3. IF YOU COULD BE A POP STAR, WHO WOULD YOU BE?
A) Jessica Simpson
B) Norah Jones
C) Jennifer Lopez
D) Amy Lee

4. WHAT'S YOUR FAVORITE HAIRSTYLE?
A) A simple braid that hangs down my back
B) Poker-straight blowout
C) Lots of big curls
D) Bed head; however it looks when I wake up in the morning

5. IF YOU'RE HITTING A PARTY, HOW LONG DOES IT TAKE YOU TO GET READY?
A) A couple of hours, but that's counting manicure, pedicure, and shopping for a new outfit
B) An hour, but there are lots of phone calls to friends beforehand to decide what I'm going to wear
C) Not long; I wear the same dark and mysterious look all the time
D) Ten minutes: a quick brush of the hair and a little sheer gloss (perhaps some mascara if it's a really big to-do)

6. IF SOMEONE SNOOPED IN YOUR MAKEUP BAG, WHAT WOULD THEY FIND?
A) Black eyeliner, black mascara, and a flyer for a concert this weekend
B) Three lip glosses, a mirror, blush, and a mini can of hairspray
C) A ponytail holder, lip balm, gum, and a mascara that's probably dried out
D) Concealer, blush, eye shadow, mascara, liner, lipstick, and an eyelash curler

7. WOULD YOU EVER LEAVE THE HOUSE WITHOUT MAKEUP ON?
A) Never. Are you insane?
B) Maybe, but I'd really miss my lip balm
C) Sure, I do it all the time
D) Sure, I've still got my nose ring

8. WHAT KIND OF NAILS DO YOU HAVE?
A) Long acrylics with different colors and designs
B) My natural ones, but I love French manicures
C) Short with a coat of clear or light polish
D) Short and naked

9. WHAT'S YOUR FAVORITE HAIR PRODUCT?
A) Shampoo
B) Hairspray
C) My straightening iron
D) Colorful hair dye

10. IF YOU COULD GO ON A DATE WITH A MUSICIAN, WOULD IT BE . . .
A) Sean "P. Diddy" Combs
B) Dave Matthews
C) Benji from Good Charlotte
D) Justin Timberlake

YOUR SCORE:

1. A=0 B=1 C=3 D=2	2. A=3 B=0 C=2 D=1	3. A=3 B=0 C=1 D=2	4. A=2 B=1 C=3 D=0	5. A=1 B=3 C=2 D=0
6. A=2 B=3 C=0 D=1	7. A=1 B=3 C=0 D=2	8. A=1 B=3 C=2 D=0	9. A=0 B=3 C=1 D=2	10. A=1 B=0 C=2 D=3

Your Score . . .

0–7, Boho Girl

YOUR MANTRA: "I'd rather save the world than buy eye shadow."
YOUR BEAUTY ROLE MODEL: *Drew Barrymore*

You're not that concerned about impressing people with your eyeliner application skills because you've got other things to do. It's not that you dislike getting glammed up, but you tend to save it for special occasions. To make your routine as easy as possible, make sure you have a great fuss-free haircut, and invest in some good skin care supplies to keep blemishes away. Remember, you don't need to pile on makeup to look your best: the newest colored mascaras add a sparkle to all eyes and a shimmery lip gloss is a must-have for every low-maintenance diva.

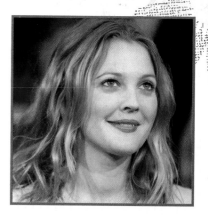

8–15, Glam Girl

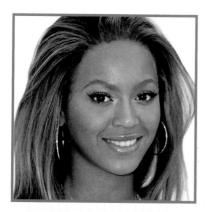

YOUR MANTRA: "I've got the walk of a supermodel and a makeup bag to match."
YOUR BEAUTY ROLE MODEL: *Beyoncé*

You are a total primping puss when it comes to your look. Your inspiration comes from beauty queens like Beyoncé, Jennifer Lopez, and Christina Aguilera. You're also a master at applying makeup—everyone turns to you for help with stuff like the smoky eye thing. Since you are fairly makeup-savvy, why not try some of the cool new retro looks, like black liquid eyeliner along the top lash line or the jewel-toned eye shadows? Remember that some of those MTV looks would look a little over-the-top in the lunchroom. The best strategy is to play up one feature at a time, such as a bright glossy mouth teamed with neutral-colored eyes in light brown or cream shadows.

16–22, Rocker Girl

YOUR MANTRA: "I like to crank up my makeup as loud as my iPod."
YOUR BEAUTY ROLE MODEL: *Amy Lee*

Rock on! You like to make a serious statement with your look, which could be described as a bunch of different things (punk, ska, rockabilly), but never middle-of-the-road. You love changing your hair (and we're not talking about a couple of golden highlights) and your makeup is anything dramatic—winged-out eyeliner, bold shadow shades, and dark lips. Why don't you try clipping on some colored hair extensions? As for makeup, check out liquid eyeliners with glitter in them so you get dramatic liner with the added bonus of a little alterna sparkle.

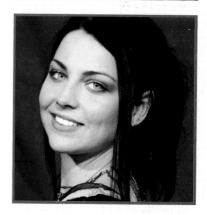

23–30, Girlie Girl

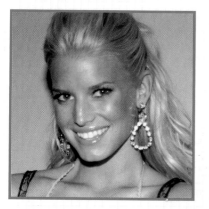

YOUR MANTRA: "I love my life and want my makeup to be rosy and romantic."
YOUR ROLE MODEL: *Jessica Simpson*

When it comes to being a girl, you love every bit of it—the fashion, the makeup, the nail polish and endless hours of trying on different hairstyles. You prefer skirts to pants (unless it's a pair of totally cute low-rise jeans) and you love all those scented lip glosses. You don't wear a ton of makeup and your favorite shades are pastels like lavender (great on all eye shades) and pale pink. You will also love all the new shimmer products on the market. Try a cream shadow and dot it on your brow bone, or a shimmery face cream dotted at the top of your cheekbones. These are easy to apply because you blend them with your fingers, and the sparkle adds a feminine touch.

QUIZ: ARE YOU STUCK IN A BEAUTY RUT?

*W*e know it's easy to slip into a bit of a routine when it comes to getting ready in the morning. While we're all for finding your style and working it, sometimes it's also fun to try something new. It can be something as easy as trying on a new lipstick shade, or something more complicated, like mastering a hair straightening technique. Just look at some of your favorite celebs–they're constantly tweaking their beauty regimens or trying something entirely new. Take this quiz to find out if you need a little helpful prodding when it comes to your beauty routine or if you're the first one on the block to switch your style.

1. WHAT'S THE MOST INTERESTING THING YOU'VE DONE WITH YOUR LOOKS RECENTLY?
A) Changed my hair part from the left to the right
B) Tried false eyelashes
C) Got a flower painted on the nail of my big toe during my pedicure

2. WHAT KIND OF JEANS DO YOU WEAR?
A) This pair that I've finally broken in after two years
B) The same hip-huggers as Jessica Simpson
C) The same brand as all my friends

3. WHERE DO YOU PUT YOUR BLUSH?
A) Well, the newest way is right in the center of my cheeks, on the apple
B) Under my cheekbones, my mom said it makes them stick out
C) The only time my cheeks look blushed is when I'm embarrassed

4. WHAT WAS THE LAST NEW PRODUCT YOU PURCHASED?
A) A colored mascara–plum looks really cool
B) A lavender eye shadow
C) A cherry lip balm

5. DO YOU KNOW HOW TO BLOW-DRY YOUR HAIR?
A) Not really, but I'm really good at twisting it up into cool styles when it's wet
B) I do it every day
C) Strictly for weddings and dances

6. IF YOU COULD COPY ANY STAR'S MAKEUP, WHOSE WOULD IT BE?
A) Pink–she always looks cool
B) Avril–I love that black eyeliner
C) Mischa Barton–she always looks pretty without looking like she tried too hard

7. HAVE YOU EVER GONE TO A COSMETICS COUNTER FOR A MAKEOVER?
A) Yeah, when I wanted to learn some new tricks
B) I'm too intimidated by those women and their perfume bottles
C) I love it—they always give out lots of freebie samples

8. WHAT'S YOUR IDEA OF LOOKING GLAM?
A) Red lipstick
B) Big curls, smoky eyes, and peach gloss
C) Wearing a little shimmer cream on my cheekbones and shoulders

9. DO YOU HAVE A SKIN CARE ROUTINE?
A) I wash and moisturize morning and night and will smear on a mask occasionally
B) My friends call my bathroom "the drugstore" because I have so many creams and things
C) I use whatever is in the bathroom

10. HOW OFTEN DO YOU GET YOUR HAIR CUT?
A) I get a trim every six months or so
B) Every couple of weeks for regular trims
C) Every three months to maintain my layers

YOUR SCORE:
1. A=3 B=1 C=2
2. A=3 B=1 C=2
3. A=1 B=2 C=3
4. A=1 B=2 C=3
5. A=2 B=1 C=3
6. A=1 B=3 C=2
7. A=2 B=3 C=1
8. A=3 B=1 C=2
9. A=2 B=1 C=3
10. A=3 B=1 C=2

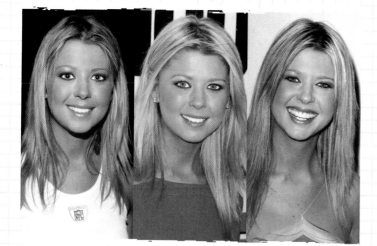

Look, it's Tara Reid in black eyeliner and a middle part . . . again, and again, and again.

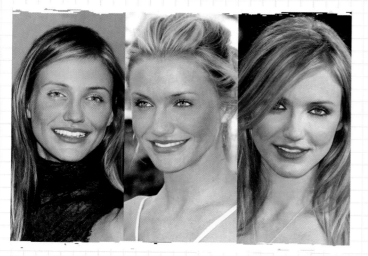

Cameron Diaz always sports her signature next-to-natural style, but she'll kick it up a notch when she needs to get glam.

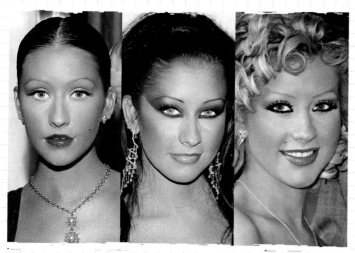

Christina Aguilera likes to change her look every five seconds, which takes serious style sass. Some makeup and hair ideas are more successful than others.

Your Score . . .
24–30, Rut Central

If you're afraid of trying something like glitter or a new haircut because you think it will look bad, think again. First of all, makeup can be washed off, so if you don't like that purple eyeliner, just ditch it. When it comes to your hair, head to a good salon for a consultation, and bring lots of pictures of styles that you could imagine having. (Also get inspired by "Our Top 10 Hairstyles" on page 102) Something as simple as a few face-framing layers or some highlights can totally transform your look.

16–23, Willing to Work It

You're totally interested in trying new things, but don't always know how to go about it. You've made minor tweaks but don't want a complete overhaul. Well, all changes don't have to be drastic. Look at your favorite stars for inspiration, but also tailor the look to suit yourself. If you love the way Gwen Stefani does her makeup, just pick out one aspect that you like and try that— red lips, liquid eyeliner, or colored shadow. Take the same approach with your hair; pick a style that you can change if you hate it. For example, long bangs can look totally rocker-girl and hang in your face, or sweet and sassy when they're brushed over to the side.

10–15, Quick-Change Artist

Whoa, we can't even keep up with you! You think of your hair as another style accessory and when it comes to makeup, anything goes. While we're totally down with trying new stuff, just make sure that everything looks good on you. Just because the newest trend is red hair doesn't mean it's right for you. Our advice? For the really drastic stuff, seek professional help (from a hairstylist or one of the women behind the cosmetics counter). Also, if you're out shopping for some new makeup, make sure to buy some stuff that you will actually wear until it runs out. Teal shadow might match those platforms you're wearing on Saturday night, but will you ever wear it again?

WHAT IT TAKES TO BE FABULOUS

*D*o you wonder how celebs manage to look good every time they leave the house? Well, what may look like an outfit that they just threw together and topped off with a little lip gloss is usually a whole lot more complicated. There's tons of preparation involved when it comes to going to a premiere or party and facing the paparazzi. It can take a whole crew of people (hair, makeup, and clothing) to get a star ready for one night out! Below, you can see just how long and how much effort and money it takes to get a celebrity like Hilary Duff red-carpet ready.

- **IF YOU'RE WONDERING** how stars always get their strands looking so fab, it's because they never have to wrestle with the blow-dryer by themselves. "Hilary's hair is in great condition," says her stylist, Colleen Conway. "I style it most of the time if she has some big event or a photo shoot."

- **TO GET HILARY'S MANE LOOKING FANTASTIC** for one night can take up to an hour of styling. Hollywood stylists are nearly always booked to show up at the celebrity's house so she doesn't have to worry about leaving the house looking undone (plus, she can get her nails done at the same time).

- **THE TYPE OF EVENT** the star is going to will determine how much the stylist will charge. For a red-carpet 'do, it's a couple hundred bucks, but for a press junket for a new movie, it can be over a thousand dollars.

- **EVER WONDER** how stars seem to go from having a short bob one day to long, flowing locks the next? "A lot of celebrities have hair extensions," says celeb stylist Robert Hallowell (he's Lucy Liu's go-to guy).

- **HAIR EXTENSIONS** can cost thousands of dollars and it takes a good stylist to help maintain the condition of the hair. Just like Hilary in this pic, tons of stars add pieces to their strands because it makes the hair look thicker. Extensions are either sewn or glued onto the hair, so there needs to be a lot of gentle maintenance to keep hair looking good.

- **CELEBS ALWAYS GET THE BEST BLING,** but it's not always because they bought it. "When you see stars walk the red carpet in tons of diamonds and other precious stones, it's almost always on loan from the jewelry store," says stylist Sherrie Kasner, who has worked with Christina Ricci, Pink, and Laura Prepon.

- **USUALLY, A STYLIST WILL BRING** the celeb a bunch of jewelry to choose from and together they'll figure out what will work best, depending on her outfit. "A lot of the really expensive pieces have to go back to the store the next day," says Kasner.

2

ALL-STAR SKIN

what you need to get glowing

QUIZ:
HOW SKIN-SAVVY ARE YOU?

Great skin can be a star's best accessory. But with so much info out there on skin care, it's hard to know what really works. Clearly there's more to taking care of your skin than just using a zit cream or eating right. Take this quiz to find out if you're in the know or scoring low when it comes to your skin.

1. WHICH IS MOST LIKELY TO CAUSE ZITS?
A) A grande vanilla latte
B) A candy bar
C) French fries

2. ASIDE FROM WRINKLES LATER IN LIFE, WHAT DOES SMOKING DO TO YOUR SKIN?
A) Aggravates acne
B) Makes it drier
C) Takes away your rosy glow

3. HOW OFTEN DO YOU NEED TO SWITCH YOUR SKIN PRODUCT?
A) Never—if it ain't broke, don't fix it
B) Twice a year
C) Whenever a new product comes out

4. WHAT PART OF YOUR SKIN IS THE MOST SENSITIVE?
A) Lips
B) Eyelids
C) Nose

5. WHEN IS THE WORST TIME TO USE A FACIAL SCRUB?
A) If your skin is really sensitive
B) If you're seeing some whiteheads
C) If your T-zone is greasier than the rest of your face

6. AT WHAT AGE IS MOST SUN DAMAGE CAUSED TO YOUR SKIN?
A) Teens
B) 20s
C) 30s

7. WHAT TYPE OF ZIT IS THE WORST?
A) A big whitehead on your cheek
B) Tons of blackheads on your nose
C) One of those painful under-the-skin bumps that you can hardly see

8. HOW DO YOU KNOW IF A MOLE ON YOUR NECK SHOULD BE CHECKED BY A DERMATOLOGIST?
A) It's over half an inch in diameter
B) It's a few different shades of brown
C) It's recently changed shape
D) Any of the above

9. WHAT'S THE BEST WAY TO GUARANTEE GOOD SKIN?
A) Become a strict vegetarian
B) Carry cleansing wipes in your book bag
C) Drink eight glasses of water a day

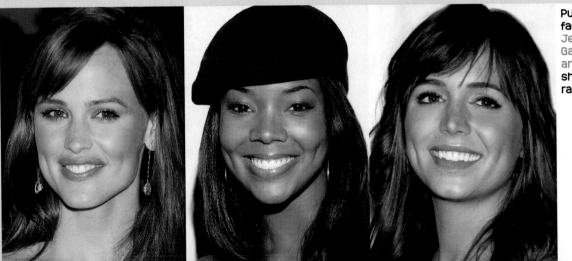

Putting their best face forward: Jennifer Garner, Gabrielle Union, and Eliza Dushku **show off their radiant skin.**

Answers:

1) A grande vanilla latte

Caffeine dehydrates you, leaving your dermis (skin) parched. This forces it into oil-producing-overdrive in an attempt to get back to normal (read: more zits). Also, since caffeine is a stimulant, it gives everything in your system a jolt, including those oil glands.

2) Takes away your rosy glow

You already know the health risks of smoking, but did you know it makes your skin look dull and lifeless? Puffing on cigarettes stops oxygen from getting to the surface of the skin so all those blood vessels that like to stay pumped up and pink get dried up. Because of this, any nicks or picked zits take longer to heal, and it is more likely that a poked pimple will leave a scar.

3) Twice a year

As tempting as it may be to try out every product that hits the shelves, it's not necessary. When it comes to skin care, all most of us need is a foaming cleanser and an oil-free moisturizer with SPF 15 in the summer. Since skin gets drier in the winter, you may need to switch to a less drying cleanser (like a cream or milk formulation) and a slightly heavier moisturizer with SPF 15—but only if you need it. A good zit cream always helps too!

4) Eyelids

The skin around the eyes is much thinner than the rest of your face and contains fewer oil glands. And with all that blinking, laughing, and finger-rubbing, this area is one of the first to show wrinkles when you get older. Also, if this sensitive skin starts to feel dry or flaky, you may want to ease up on the eye makeup. Finally, always remember to remove all mascara and liner with an eye makeup remover before cleansing the rest of your face before bed.

5) If you're seeing some whiteheads

Since scrubs contain small granules that remove pore-clogging dead skin, they can be too harsh on acne. If you have a whitehead on your face, the grains could cause you to rub the top off of the pimple and spread the bacteria from the zit across your face, which could lead to more breakouts.

6) Teens

The majority of sun damage happens during the first 15 years of life. There's also more than enough data to show that single sunburns from childhood will come back to haunt you (i.e., wrinkles, brown spots, and possibly worse . . .). These days it's so easy to keep skin protected without major effort by using a tinted moisturizer or foundation with an SPF for everyday coverage. However, if you're doing some serious summer sun time, apply a sunscreen with at least an SPF of 15 to your face.

7) One of those painful under-the-skin bumps that you can hardly see

While the whiteheads and blackheads may look much worse, these bumps (called cystic acne) are more serious and don't respond to over-the-counter treatments. Cystic acne forms much deeper in the skin when oil glands clog up, and it is best treated with oral medications like tetracycline, or in severe cases, Accutane®. But, just like other members of the acne family, these painful bumps should never be picked—they can rupture under the skin and cause a larger infection.

8) Any of the above

The general rule of thumb when it comes to moles is this: If you're not sure, go to a doctor and have it checked. Just as you go for your annual checkup, you should do the same with a dermatologist if you have ANY suspicious-looking moles. Also, keep an eye on them yourself. If you notice any changes (in shape, color, or size) make an appointment with a dermatologist immediately.

9) Carry cleansing wipes in your book bag

We've all heard that junk food gives you spots, but it's not true. While it does help to eat nutritious stuff like fruits and vegetables because your body gets those much-needed vitamins and minerals, a candy bar isn't going to make you break out. What will make you break out is airborne grease and bacteria. Another habit that exacerbates acne is touching your face, since your fingers carry a lot of pimple-causing bacteria. So if you're prone to pimples, pick up some of those cleansing wipes from the drug store and use one whenever your face feels greasy.

QUIZ: WHAT'S YOUR SKIN TYPE?

he first step to achieving flawless movie-star skin like Halle Berry's or Jennifer Lopez's is to figure out what type of skin you have so you can treat it right. Without knowing that bit of skinfo, no cleansers, moisturizers, or pimple products will do you any good, because you won't know which ones to use or how to use them.

Just because a product keeps Jessica Simpson's gorgeous face looking poreless doesn't mean it will do the same for Missy Elliott—or you. Copying someone else's skin care routine could even make your skin worse! So, before applying another drop of lotion, take this quiz to figure out what your skin is—dry, oily, or combination—then get the scoop on what you need to do to get picture-perfect skin.

1. WASH YOUR FACE WITH A GENTLE CLEANSER, PAT DRY, AND DON'T APPLY ANY PRODUCTS FOR 15 MINUTES. YOUR SKIN FEELS:

A) Kind of dry on your cheeks, but a little slick on your forehead, nose, and chin

B) Oily all over

C) Tight and even a little irritated and itchy

2. TAKE A CLOSE LOOK AT YOUR FACE—NOSE TO REFLECTED NOSE AT THE MIRROR (OR USE A MAGNIFYING MIRROR). WHERE ARE YOUR PORES MOST NOTICEABLE?

A) Forehead, nose, and chin, forming a straight line down your face

B) Everywhere!

C) Nowhere, really

3. NOW TAKE A LOOK AT THE SIZE OF YOUR PORES— WHERE DO YOU SEE THE BIGGEST PORES? THEY LOOK:

A) Big on your nose and chin, but small on your cheeks

B) Kind of large all over

C) Virtually invisible or at least very tiny

4. WHEN ZITS POP UP, THEY TEND TO APPEAR:

A) In the center of your face—on your forehead and chin as well as all around your nose

B) All over!

C) Mostly on your chin, but every once in a while, they pop up in other spots, like your forehead and cheeks

5. WHEN YOU GET ZITS, THEY LOOK LIKE:

A) Either dome-shaped red bumps (a.k.a. your standard, run-of-the-mill pimple) or whiteheads (a little grosser than your everyday red bump and so hard to resist popping)

B) Everything from dome-shaped red bumps to white-capped monsters to painful mountainlike cysts that seem to last forever

C) Either dome-shaped red bumps or tiny, hard red bumps that appear only on your cheeks. (Pssst! These aren't really zits, but we'll get to that later)

6. WASH YOUR HANDS AND THEN RUN A FINGER OVER YOUR FACE. THE TEXTURE FEELS:

A) A little bumpy on your forehead, nose, and chin, but smooth on your cheeks

B) Basically bumpy and uneven all over

C) Flaky and dry, and maybe a little bumpy on your cheeks

7. YOUR LIPS USUALLY FEEL:

A) Sometimes dry. You never know from day to day when you'll need to use lip balm so you always stash some in your purse

B) Just right. They are always soft and supple

C) Dry and chapped. You apply lip balm a million times a day

8. WHEN YOU STAND BACK FROM THE MIRROR, YOUR OVERALL COMPLEXION LOOKS:

A) Shiny on the T-zone, around your nose and on your chin

B) Shiny all over—your forehead, nose, cheeks, and chin

C) Not shiny at all—instead, your skin looks flat

9. AFTER YOU WASH YOUR HAIR IN THE MORNING, YOUR SCALP STARTS TO FEEL GREASY:

A) After a day

B) By lunch!

C) It can go as long as three or four days before the greasies set in, but you probably like to suds up every other day anyway

10. WHEN YOU WAKE UP IN THE MORNING, YOUR FACE CRAVES:

A) A washing with water and cleanser

B) A big-time wipe down with astringent wash or pads

C) Moisturizer, ASAP

Your answers to perfect skin

HERE'S YOUR SKINFORMATION, WITH SKIN CARE TIPS FROM KATIE RODAN, MD, DERMATOLOGIST TO SUCH STARS AS BRITNEY SPEARS, JESSICA SIMPSON, AND RENÉE ZELLWEGER.

If you picked mostly As . . .
You have combination skin.

DILEMMA: YOUR T-ZONE, WHICH INCLUDES YOUR FOREHEAD, NOSE, AND CHIN, IS OILY WHILE THE EYE AREA, CHEEKS, AND NECK ARE DRY AND POSSIBLY FLAKY.

Game plan:
MORNING: "Wash your face, focusing mainly on the T-zone, with a gel-based cleansing fluid or glycerin bar," recommends Rodan. Rinse thoroughly with lukewarm water and pat dry. Apply an oil-absorbing lotion to your T-zone, then cover your entire face with an oil-free sunscreen with SPF 15 or higher. Stash blotting sheets in your bag, so you can blot away any greasies that pop up throughout the day.

NIGHT: Wash with lukewarm water and a gel-based cleanser that contains salicylic acid, again focusing on the mid-section of your face; "the salicylic acid will help unplug the pores on your T-zone," says Rodan. Rinse with lukewarm water, pat dry, and apply a lotion that contains salicylic acid to your T-zone and an oil-free moisture lotion to the rest of your face, primarily your cheeks.

ONCE A WEEK: To dry up the oil in your greasiest areas, treat just your T-zone to an oil-absorbing clay mask.

MAKEUP TIP: Stick to oil-free concealers and liquid foundations, which won't clog pores.

If you picked mostly Bs . . .
You have oily skin.

DILEMMA: YOUR OIL GLANDS ARE IN OVERDRIVE, SO SKIN IS SHINY AND PORES ARE CLOGGED, CAUSING BLACKHEADS, WHITEHEADS, AND PIMPLES.

Game plan:
MORNING: Wash your skin with a gel-based cleanser that contains salicylic acid, to help strip away oil and unplug clogged pores. Use lukewarm water to wash and then gently pat your face dry with a towel. Follow up with a toner that also contains salicylic acid and top with an oil-absorbing lotion, applied all over your face. Finish with an oil-free gel (not lotion) sunscreen of SPF 15 or higher (gel-based sunscreens look clear, not white). "Gel-based sunscreens contain a bit of alcohol, which will help keep oil under control," explains Rodan. Tote around oil-blotting sheets, so you can wipe away oil during the day.

NIGHT: At night, wash with the same cleanser and lukewarm water, pat dry with a towel, and follow up with the salicylic acid toner. Finish with a lotion that also contains salicylic acid.

ONCE A WEEK: Apply an oil-absorbing clay mask in a thin layer all over your face to dry up the grease and keep it under control.

MAKEUP TIP: Foundations and concealers that contain salicylic acid will help fend off greasy skin while covering imperfections.

If you picked mostly Cs . . .
You have dry skin.

DILEMMA: YOUR UNDERPRODUCTIVE OIL GLANDS LEAVE YOUR SKIN TIGHT AND FLAKY AND, IN SOME CASES, COVERED IN TINY, HARD BUMPS (USUALLY FOUND ON CHEEKS).

Game plan:
MORNING: Wash with a mild soap-free cleanser that contains no alcohol. Use lukewarm water to wash and then gently pat your face dry with a towel. Cover your face with an oil-free moisturizer that is for normal to dry skin. Finish with an oil-free, SPF 15 or higher sunscreen.

NIGHT: Wash your face with the same mild soap-free cleanser, rinse with lukewarm water, and pat dry with a towel. Exfoliate dry patches with a lotion that contains glycolic acid, applying it only to dry and flaky spots. Top it with an oil-free moisturizer, applied over your entire face.

ONCE A WEEK: Moisturize your skin with a hydrating face mask to make it feel soft and less irritated.

MAKEUP TIP: Choose only creamy foundation formulations and moisturizing lipsticks.

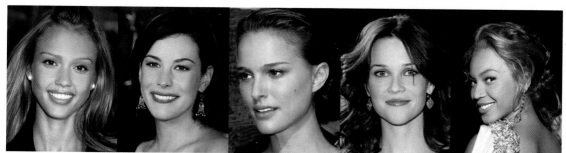

The fab five:
Jessica Alba, Liv Tyler, Natalie Portman, Reese Witherspoon, and Beyoncé have the best skin in the business

STAR TREATMENTS

*O*ne of the ways celebs stay looking so camera-ready and confident is by making the time to schedule regular spa treatments. While we can't book you a free airline ticket to Los Angeles to check out the pampering procedures yourself, we did snag the beauty pros and have them give us their at-home versions of these sought-after skin and hair treatments.

DREW BARRYMORE'S BLEMISH BUSTER

When Drew Barrymore isn't off on location shooting another block-buster movie, she loves to get facials from Sonya Dakar, one of the most sought-after skin specialists in Hollywood. To keep her skin clear if she can't get in for a pampering, Drew stocks up on Sonya's Drying Potion, which works overnight to dry out any body blemishes. Here's how to make your own all-star mix:

What You'll Need
❑ MIXING BOWL
❑ WHISK
❑ COTTON SWABS

Ingredients
❑ 1 SMALL PACKET DRY YEAST
❑ 8 OZ. SPRING WATER
❑ 1 LEMON WEDGE

To Mix
Pour the yeast packet into a bowl. Add water, a few drops at a time, whisking well after each H_2O addition. Keep adding water until the mixture turns into a medium thick paste (usually about 2 tablespoons of water). Squeeze a few drops of lemon juice into the mix and stir again.

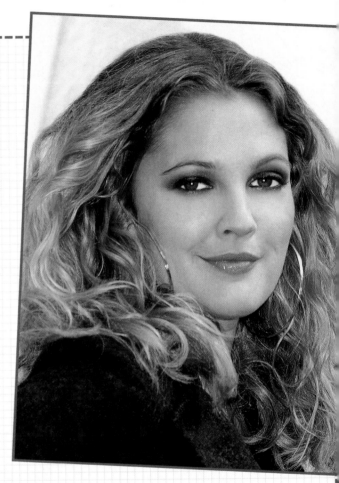

★ IRRITATION ALERT!
Before you go crazy smearing your skin and hair in these delicious beauty treats, it's a good idea to do an allergy spot test. To do this, just apply a small amount of the mixture on the inside of your lower arm. Let it sit there for a couple of hours and if there's no reaction, feel free to apply the product elsewhere. Note: To avoid a big bowl of mixture that you can't use (if you do have a reaction), cut the recipe in half if you want to test it out.

To Use
Wash your face and pat dry with a towel. Dot the mixture on any breakouts using a cotton swab. Wait 30 seconds for it to dry. Wash off in the morning using warm water and a cleanser. Tip: this mixture is also safe for body acne on shoulders or chest.

How Long It Lasts
You can keep this mixture in your bathroom in an airtight container for one week.

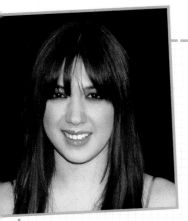

MICHELLE BRANCH'S BEAUTIFYING FACE SCRUB

Being on the road and touring can cause skin to become dehydrated and clog pores, so whenever Michelle Branch swings through LA for a concert or a red-carpet appearance, she always stops by Enessa Aromatherapy for a facial from Michelle Ornstein. She likes an exfoliating treatment that scrubs off dead skin and curbs blemishes. Here's how to make your own clear-skin scrub. The almonds and oatmeal help get rid of dead skin cells that can clog up pores and cause breakouts; the honey and lavender are antibacterial and moisturizing (you may be tempted to eat it, but don't!).

What You'll Need
- ❏ FOOD PROCESSOR
- ❏ MIXING BOWL
- ❏ MIXING SPOON
- ❏ TOWELS

Ingredients
- ❏ HANDFUL ALMONDS
- ❏ 1 TBSP. OATMEAL
- ❏ 1 TBSP. HONEY
- ❏ 1 DROP LAVENDER ESSENTIAL OIL
  (FOUND AT HEALTH FOOD STORES)

To Mix
Throw the almonds into the food processor and mix at high speed for 10 seconds or until nuts turn into a powder (kind of like sand). Pour almond powder into a bowl. Add all the remaining ingredients to the almond powder and mix with a spoon until it turns into a paste.

To Use
Wash your face with your normal cleanser and pat dry with a towel. Scoop up a handful of the scrub, rub both hands together to distribute the mask evenly, then gently scrub the skin using a circular motion. Avoid the delicate skin around the eye area. Rinse off with warm water after 20 seconds, pat face dry with a towel, and admire your beautiful skin in the mirror! Apply a light moisturizer if skin feels dry.

How Long It Lasts
Since your skin doesn't need to be scrubbed two days in a row and the mixture could go bad, toss any leftovers as soon as you are done.

KIRSTEN DUNST'S MAGIC MOISTURE MASK

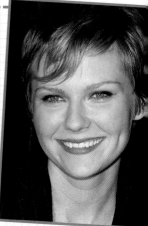

This too-cute star is a regular at LA's Sonya Dakar Skin Clinic, where she gets facials from Sonya herself. Kirsten knows that one of the best tricks to keep skin glowing (especially in warm climates like California) is to keep it moisturized. While Kirsten stocks up on products while she is at Sonya's clinic, we snagged a mask recipe that you can make yourself. This mask is great if your skin is dry, like after a day at the pool or the beach, thanks to hydrating and soothing ingredients like aloe vera gel and honey.

What You'll Need
- ❏ MIXING BOWL
- ❏ FORK
- ❏ MIXING SPOON
- ❏ TOWELS

Ingredients
- ❏ ½ MEDIUM-SIZE AVOCADO, PEELED AND PITTED
- ❏ 2 TBSP. ALOE VERA GEL
  (AT DRUG OR HEALTH FOOD STORES)
- ❏ 1 TBSP. HONEY
- ❏ 2 TBSP. PLAIN OLD-FASHIONED OATMEAL (NOT INSTANT)
- ❏ 1 TSP. GRAPESEED OIL
  (AT GROCERY OR HEALTH FOOD STORES)

To Mix
Using a fork, mash the avocado in the bowl until it is semi-smooth but still has a few lumps. Add the aloe vera gel to the avocado and mix together thoroughly. Mix in the rest of the ingredients and stir until they're totally blended.

To Use
Wash your face and pat dry with a towel. Scoop out small handfuls of the mask and smear it onto your face. Keep applying until you've covered all the skin on your face (avoiding the delicate skin around your eyes) in a thickish layer. Next, chill out for 15 minutes while the mask absorbs into your face. When the time is up, rinse the mask off using warm water and then pat skin dry with a towel.

How Long It Lasts
With fresh ingredients like avocado, any leftovers of this mask should be tossed right after you are done.

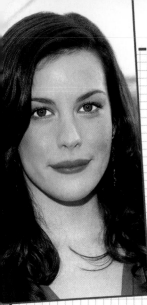

LIV TYLER'S SHINY HAIR MASK

When she's in LA, Liv Tyler always stops by Tina Cassaday's Beverly Hills salon for some tress treats. Cassaday is known for whipping up fruity concoctions that condition damaged hair, add vibrant shine, and smell terrific. One of her newest products (and one of Liv's faves) is a banana conditioner that's packed with all the vitamins and minerals your hair needs to stay strong and shiny.

What You'll Need
- ❑ BLENDER
- ❑ SPATULA
- ❑ MIXING BOWL
- ❑ TOWEL
- ❑ SHOWER CAP
- ❑ WIDE-TOOTHED COMB

Ingredients
- ❑ ½ CUP PINT PURIFIED WATER
- ❑ ½ BANANA, PEELED
- ❑ 1 TBSP. PLAIN YOGURT
- ❑ 1 TSP. HONEY
- ❑ ¼ CANTALOUPE, PEELED AND SEEDED
- ❑ 1 TBSP. CONDENSED MILK
- ❑ 1 TSP. WHEAT GERM OIL (FOUND AT HEALTH FOOD STORES)

To Mix
Put all the ingredients in the blender and blend for 10 seconds using the medium setting. Pour the mixture into a bowl, using a spatula to scoop all of the mask out the blender.

To Use
Put a towel across your shoulders to avoid any spills on your clothes. Take some of the mixture in your hand and apply to a big section of dry hair, starting from the roots and working your way down to the ends. Do this until your whole head is covered with the mask. Twist up the ends of your hair and lightly pin them to the top of your head and then slip on the shower cap (this stops drips as well as helps the conditioner to really penetrate the hair). Leave on for a minimum of 45 minutes before rinsing off with warm water. Use a light shampoo to get rid of any food remnants. When you're finished, detangle locks with a wide-tooth comb and let hair air-dry so it will feel super soft.

How Long It Lasts
With fruit and yogurt as key ingredients, any remnants of this tress treat should be tossed when you're done.

LUCY LIU'S BODY-BOOSTING HAIR TREATMENT

This *Charlie's Angels* star has some of the shiniest strands in Hollywood. Her stylist Robert Hallowell, also known as The Kitchen Beautician, is always whipping up different concoctions to pamper her hair with natural ingredients. One of his favorites is this avocado mask which adds body and shine as the avocado is super-moisturizing and the lemon helps to bring out hair's natural shine.

What You'll Need
- ❑ MIXING BOWL
- ❑ MIXING SPOON
- ❑ FORK
- ❑ SIEVE
- ❑ TOWELS
- ❑ SHOWER CAP
- ❑ WIDE-TOOTH COMB

Ingredients:
- ❑ 4 TBSP. LEMON JUICE (if you are using freshly squeezed lemon juice, pour it through a sieve first to eliminate pulp)
- ❑ 1 MEDIUM-SIZED AVOCADO, PEELED, PITTED, AND SLICED
- ❑ 1 TBSP. BLACKSTRAP MOLASSES

To Mix
Put the sliced avocado in the bowl and use a fork to mash it up until it's smushed but still a bit lumpy. Add the lemon juice and the molasses and mix with a spoon.

To Use
Put a towel across your shoulders to avoid any spills on your clothes. Scoop the mixture out of the bowl and, grabbing a large section of dry hair, smear it onto strands, starting at the scalp and working your way down in sections until all your hair is covered with the mask. Lightly pin any loose ends to your head and slip on a shower cap; wait 20 minutes so the avocado oil can really penetrate the hair shaft. When the time is up, hop into the shower and rinse off the mask with warm water, then use a light shampoo to get rid of any food remnants. Detangle hairusing a wide-toothed comb and let it air-dry so it will feel super soft.

How Long It Lasts
With quick-to-spoil ingredients like avocado, any remains of this mask should be tossed when you're done.

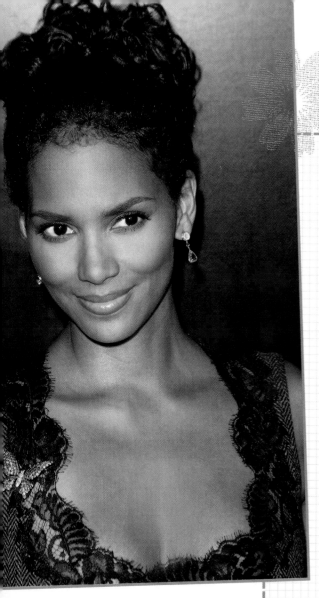

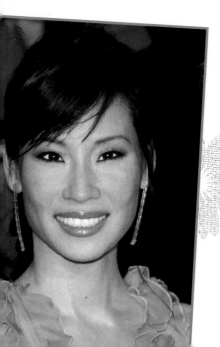

HALLE BERRY'S PEACHY KEEN BODY SCRUB

Halle Berry is known for always looking top-to-toe flawless and is just as conscientious about the skin on her body as she is about the skin on her face. She makes regular appointments to come in to Kinara Spa in West Hollywood for treatments from owner Olga Lorencin-Northrup and even purchases her line of products to use at home. Lorencin-Northrup created this at-home recipe for an amazing peach scrub that you can use on your body. Not only does it smell delicious, but the sugar scrubs off flaky, dry skin while the peaches give you a vitamin C fix. This is a perfect scrub to apply in the evening before you go to bed.

What You'll Need
- ❏ BLENDER
- ❏ MEDIUM-SIZE PLASTIC BOWL
- ❏ MIXING SPOON
- ❏ TWO TOWELS

Ingredients
- ❏ 2 MEDIUM OR 3 SMALL PEACHES, PEELED, PITTED, AND SLICED INTO MEDIUM-SIZED SLICES
- ❏ 1 CUP BROWN SUGAR
- ❏ 2 CUPS ALMOND OIL (AT HEALTH FOOD STORES)

To Mix
Put the peach slices in the blender. Blend on high for 10 seconds. Scoop out the peach mixture into a bowl; add the brown sugar and the almond oil. Using a spoon, stir the mixture until it is blended.

To Use
Take the bowl with you into the bathroom and hop into the shower, but don't turn on the water. Apply handfuls of the scrub to your arms and legs, rubbing it in using an up-and-down motion (this scrub is too grainy to use on your face). You'll know you're done when the sugar dissolves. Rinse off any remnants with warm water but avoid using soap, as that will wash away all the good ingredients. When you're finished rinsing, gently blot skin dry. Since your skin will feel so soft, you can skip body lotion.

How Long It Lasts
Since it contains fresh fruit, any leftovers should be tossed immediately after use.

SENSATIONAL SKIN

Still not sure what's the best thing for your skin, or why your face can look flawless one day, but not the next? Skin queen Sonya Dakar, who has pampered the pores of Gwyneth Paltrow and Brittany Murphy, and Dr. Norman Leaf, who counts Courteney Cox Arquette as a fan of his skin care products, answers your most pressing questions about how to get gorgeous skin, as well as why your own face has the occasional freak-out and what you can do about it.

Q. Why is it that your skin starts going nuts the minute you become a teenager? What is happening inside your body that makes it break out?

A. "When you become a teenager your body goes through a lot of hormonal changes," says Dr. Leaf. "There is an increase in the hormone estrogen in girls and testosterone in boys." These hormones contribute to a boost of the oil production in the skin. Although your body is constantly shedding old skin cells to reveal a new layer of fresh cells underneath, with all of that extra lube on your face, dead skin cells get stuck on the skin's surface, which leads to pores getting clogged. The end result is either a blackhead or a whitehead.

Q. I feel like I eat fairly healthfully and always wash my face before bed. My friend, however, lives on fast food and even hits the pillow with her makeup on sometimes. I have zits and she doesn't. What gives?

A. As important as it is to take good care of your skin, whether or not you get acne is largely up to your parents. Just like genetics decide whether or not you're going to get Dad's blue eyes or Mom's brown ones, it can also decide how much acne you're going to have (bummer, we know). However, if you look back at your folk's yearbook pics and see that their complexions are less than perfect, at least you'll know what you're up against. "I recommend the moment a teenager starts getting acne that he or she can't control with regular over-the-counter products, that they go to a dermatologist," says Dr. Leaf. "The longer you wait the worse it will become." Also, there are so many more choices these days when it comes to skin care that, if your parents didn't have perfect skin, chances are there's a product that can help.

Emily Van Kamp seems to have the good skin genes.

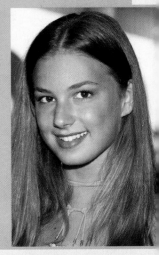

Q. What is the #1 thing that celebrities do to keep their skin looking fabulous?

A. Stay out of the sun. "I had one young actress come to me and I ended up turning her away because she wouldn't stop going to tanning booths and the beach," says Dakar. If you need proof of what the sun does to your skin, just compare a section of your bod that never sees the sun (like your belly) to a section that does (your forearm) and note the difference in texture. Most stars are pretty sun-savvy—either they prefer to stick with their natural fair-skinned tone, like Nicole Kidman or Scarlett Johansson, or they're like Christina Aguilera, who gets her bronze-Betty look from self-tanner instead of hours spent in the sun. The easiest way to make sunscreen a part of your daily beauty regimen is to buy either a moisturizer or a tinted moisturizer that contains an SPF. "For the face, I suggest nothing less than SPF 15," says Dakar. Also, don't forget other sun-sensitive areas like the earlobes and, if you part your hair, keep in mind that your exposed scalp can also be burned.

Scarlett likes her look soft and pretty.

Q. Do celebrities eat anything special to make their skin look so good?

A. While we know that eating chocolate isn't going to give you acne, that doesn't mean you have free reign to go and devour the whole drive-thru and expect a glowy complexion. "It's important to get the right vitamins for your skin," says Dakar. For teen clients she always suggests zinc (found in meat, milk, and beans), vitamin C (citrus fruits), and flaxseed oil (can be bought at the health food store and drizzled over a salad). Zinc and vitamin C work to protect the skin and strengthen it. Flaxseed oil actually has the power to thin the blood in your skin a little bit so pores may not get as clogged. All three of these help the skin to heal more quickly, which, if you've ever picked a zit, you know can take a while. "Also, don't forget to drink water," adds Dakar, "without it your skin can look dry and tired." Not that you need to go on a crazy diet to have good skin, just remember to balance out the fries with lots of natural stuff like fruits and veggies—these naturally contain a lot of the vitamins and minerals your body needs, plus, they're more filling than popping a pill!

Jennifer Lopez steals the show with flawless features.

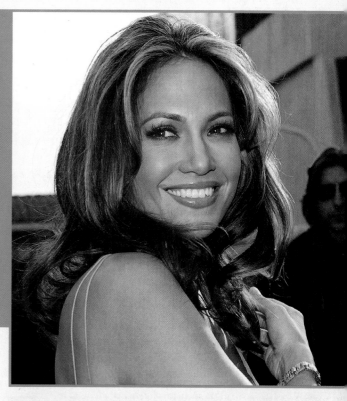

Q. How do celebs always look so fresh-faced and flawless when they're walking the red carpet?

A. Good question. First of all, don't forget that celebs probably climb straight out of an air-conditioned limo, walk the red carpet for 10 minutes, and then head into an air-conditioned building. Also, they have a few tricks up their sleeve when it comes to treating the skin. "The are tons of oil-absorbing moisturizers on the market, that can hyrate the skin while still absorbing some of the extra grease on your oilier parts like forehead and nose," says Dakar. Also, if you are prone to looking a little greasy, avoid wearing too much makeup because it will just get cakey. Hollywood makeup artist Agostina for Cloutier, who has made up such stars as Jennifer Love Hewitt and Mischa Barton, likes to use an oil-free liquid foundation and loose powder. "A lot of stars don't wear huge amounts of makeup because it always look obvious, " she says. "It's not supposed to look like you're wearing foundation, it's supposed to look like you have great skin!"

Jennifer Freeman always glows on the red carpet.

Q. I'm only 15 and I already have dark circles around my eyes. What is going on? It makes me look like I'm tired even when I've had a good night's sleep.

A. "Since the skin under the eyes is so thin, a lot of times the darker discoloration is because you can see the dark blood vessels through that part of the skin," says Dr. Leaf. Another reason is your skin tone. And again, blame genetics. If you have olive or darker skin, you can end up with more pigment under the eye area than on the rest of your face. An easy way to tell if this is you is if the circle is more of a dark brown (darker than your skin tone). While it's difficult to make these disappear, taking care of your body can always help. If you smoke, quit now, since puffing restricts the blood vessels, which can exaggerate circles. Also, stimulants like coffee that can stop you from getting a good night sleep aren't so great.

On the bright side, it's easy to hide dark circles with concealer. Just pick a shade that's the same shade as the skin on the rest of your face. We think the easiest formulations to apply under the eye area are the thicker formulations (they come in a tube like a lipstick) because you can just put a dot in the lower inner corner of your eye and then pat it into the skin with a clean finger. When you're applying concealer, you don't have to sweep it underneath the whole eye, apply it only on the inner half of your under-eye area and then blend. If you go all the way, you'll look like a raccoon. Also, if you don't want those dark circles to look darker, avoid wearing a lot of dark eyeliners and mascaras on the lower eyelid.

TOP 10 WAYS TO ZAP A ZIT

There's no escaping zits–everybody gets them! It's amazing how a zit (or two or three) can ruin an otherwise perfect morning. Even celebs can't escape the dreaded breakout! (In case you were wondering why there are no celebs on this page? That's because superstars know how to dodge the photographers until the darn things disappear!)

Lucky for all of us, there are ways to head a pimple off at the pass as well as ways to treat breakouts that have already made their unwelcome appearance. Below are our top 10 best solutions for dealing with spotty situations, straight from dermatologists-to-the-stars Kathy Fields, MD and Michael Gold, MD.

1. KEEP YOUR SKIN MOISTURIZED.
"While it may seem like a good idea to suck out every last drop of oil from your skin by bagging the use of a moisturizer or overloading it with drying acne medications, it's really counterproductive," says Fields. When your skin is too dry, something called the androgen hormone is likely to kick into overdrive and work like mad to compensate for the dry

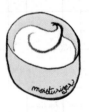

conditions, producing tons of sebum (a.k.a. oil) to compensate. This is likely to lead to clogged pores, and even more likely, the dreaded zit. Plus, the ones you already have will look worse. If you've got oily skin, make sure you're using an oil-free moisturizer or gel rather than a cream, and apply it every morning.

2. EXFOLIATE TO STOP A ZIT BEFORE IT STARTS.
When sebum (also known as oil) is doing its job well, it carries dead skin cells to the surface of the skin so they can be washed away. Unfortunately for us, sometimes pores become clogged and the dead skin cells stay put inside of them, trapping oil and bacteria. As this gunk builds up, it forms a zit. "Exfoliation is the process of removing dead skin cells before they have a chance to clog up your pores," says Fields. There are two ways to exfoliate: 1) physical scrubs and 2) chemical exfoliators. Use physical scrubs that have perfectly spherical beads to gently remove dead skin cells, oil, and bacteria (scrubs with jagged beads, like apricot scrubs, are harsh and can irritate your face). This type of scrub should not be used if you have tons of pimples spread over your face, since it could irritate them. Chemical exfoliators use their different chemical bases to remove the dead skin—like retinoids, beta hydroxy acids, or alpha hydroxy acids. They come in different formulations, such as lotions and gels, and remove dead skin cells without scrubbing. You can get them at the drugstore. Follow directions on the bottle or tube for use.

3. SEE A DERMATOLOGIST.
Doctors have lots of tricks to banish pimples. They can also prescribe stronger acne medications than you can get at the store, like topical antibiotics. Plus, "derms are now zapping zits with lasers that penetrate the skin and photo-destroy acne-forming bacteria," says Dr. Gold. Downside: the treatments do not work overnight; typically it takes about four weeks to see results, and with two visits to the doctor a week, the process can be expensive. Upside: laser treatments can get rid of zits for a long time.

4. STOP STRESSING.
Every time you freak out over a guy, a test, or your drama with family and friends, "your hormones fluctuate like mad, which leads to oil production, which can lead to clogged pores, which can lead to the dreaded zit," says Dr. Gold. So, once a day, try to take a few deep breaths, chill out, and take some quiet time for yourself to relieve stress.

5. USE SUN PROTECTION.
"Ideally, pick something with an SPF of 15 or higher," says Fields. There are non-oily formulations made especially for faces. We know, a tan can disguise zits, and being out in the sun even seems like it dries them up. But, in reality, the sun makes the zits you have worse and is likely to cause more to pop up. The sun dries out your skin, and your oil glands go into overdrive to compensate (just like we explained in reason #1). In essence, your face turns into one big oil slick and the zits you have get bigger and ready to pop.

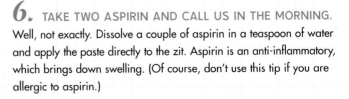

6. TAKE TWO ASPIRIN AND CALL US IN THE MORNING.
Well, not exactly. Dissolve a couple of aspirin in a teaspoon of water and apply the paste directly to the zit. Aspirin is an anti-inflammatory, which brings down swelling. (Of course, don't use this tip if you are allergic to aspirin.)

7. TREAT A ZIT WITH AN ON-THE-SPOT ACNE TREATMENT, WHICH CONTAINS INGREDIENTS THAT HELP REDUCE INFLAMMATION. "To dry up a zit, try benzoyl peroxide 2.5 percent or salicylic acid 0.5 percent," says Fields. Don't use anything stronger than 2.5 percent or you may dry your skin out too much and cause a slew of other problems. The key here is not to go nuts with a product; simply dab a small amount on the zit, and get on with your life.

8. USE AN ACNE-FIGHTING FACE MASK. Once a week, treat your skin to a mask that helps fight off clogged pores or breakouts. You have a couple of choices: "Clay" masks will help suck up excess oil in your skin and unplug clogged pores. "Medicated" masks containing benzoyl peroxide (just like on-the-spot treatments) are another good choice to help heal existing pimples. For the best results, alternate between a clay and medicated mask every other week. Make sure you leave the mask on for the exact time recommended in the instructions on the box, or you can irritate your skin. (These masks are both fine to use when you have a breakout; in fact, they will help heal the zits.)

9. SHRINK A PIMPLE WITH AN ICE PACK. Since ice can be irritating, cover a few cubes with a washcloth, then hold the ice pack against your pimple for about 10 minutes. It's the same principle as icing a sprained ankle to keep the swelling down.

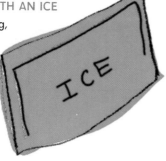

10. USE EYEDROPS TO MAKE THE REDNESS LOOK LESS NOTICEABLE IN AN INSTANT. Eyedrops are made to reduce the redness in your eyes, but they will do the same for a pimple. A couple of drops should do the trick.

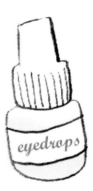

★ ZIT PICKING 101

Pop a pimple only as the very, very LAST RESORT! Since we know you are going to do this anyway, we might as well tell you how to do it to cause the least possible damage, if you absolutely, positively must. Listen up: popping will only work on a pimple that has a white cap, not those big, bumpy, pink ones. If you try to pick those (the ones that actually hurt), you will make them much, much worse. If you have the right kind of zit, this is what you have to do: Wash your face and hands with a gentle cleanser and lukewarm water, to rid your skin of bacteria and open the pores a bit. Wet a clean washcloth with warm water (previously used washcloths can be breeding grounds for bacteria, which can invade your skin and cause more pimples). Wrap a corner of the washcloth around each of your pointer fingers and squeeze the pimple very gently, so the white pus squirts out. After you are finished, top the popped pimple with benzoyl peroxide, which will keep bacteria at bay. WARNING: Popping zits can lead to enlarged pores, red marks that take forever to go away, and even scars.

PIMPLE COVER-UP

The best way to cover up a pimple so it looks natural is to use a cream or stick foundation that matches your skin with a yellow undertone. Finding a shade that is a yellowish version of your exact skin tone is really important because it will be better at concealing a pink pimple—just think, if you put a pink tone on top of something that is already pink, it will look pinker, right? No lighter, no darker, or it will draw more attention to the zit. (For more info on choosing foundation and concealer colors and formulas, check out "Getting Gorgeous" on page 44). Don't smear the foundation all over your face, just apply it to your zits. Here's how:

1. After cleansing your skin with a gentle cleanser, apply an oil-free moisturizer over your entire face to create a smooth surface.

2. Using a small, pointed concealer brush or a clean finger, gently tap foundation directly onto the center of the zit until it fades away. Don't blend the foundation in too much or you will just wipe away the product.

3. Set the foundation so it stays put all day with a touch of either loose or pressed translucent powder (for info on how to set powder, see "Getting Gorgeous" on page 44).

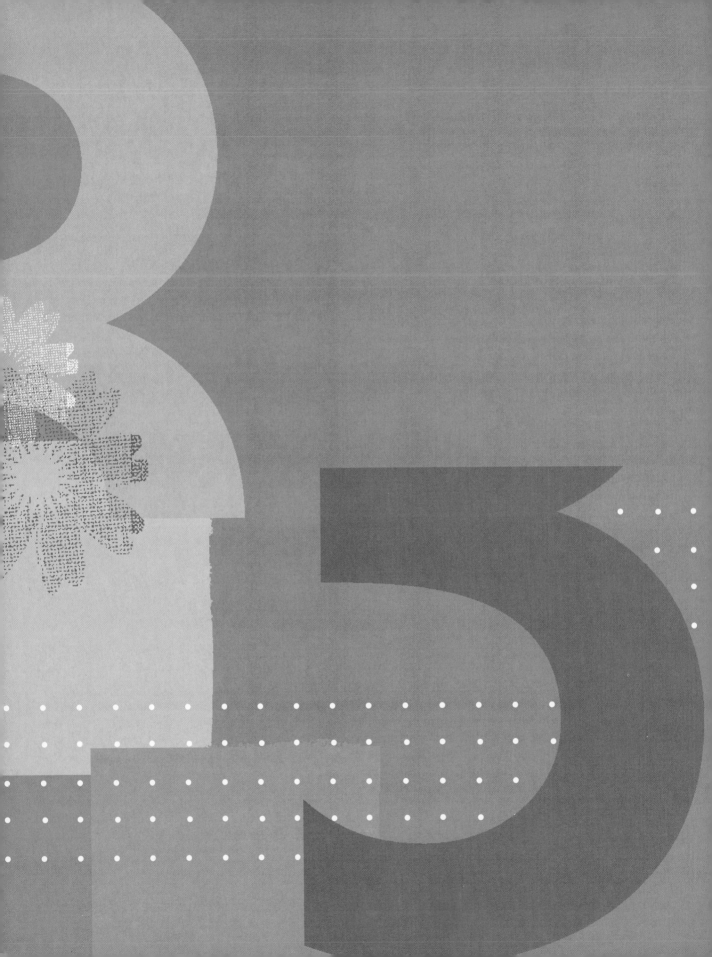

chapter three

READY FOR YOUR CLOSE-UP?

must-have makeup secrets from pros in the know

QUIZ: WHO IS YOUR MAKEUP MUSE?

*W*hether you're into mucho makeup like Christina Aguilera or a minimalist approach like Hilarie Burton, there's a celeb look out there that we know you're dying to copy. Once you figure out whose look you love, feel free to take it, tweak it, and make it all your own. Answer the questions below to see what should be in your makeup bag.

1. HOW OFTEN DO YOU WEAR MAKEUP?

A) Every day

B) Maybe a little during the day and something fun on weekends

C) Only if I go out, and even then I like to keep it simple

2. WHEN NEW MAKEUP TRENDS COME OUT, YOU:

A) Think they're great for other people, but not for you

B) Try one that isn't too crazy

C) Immediately rush out and buy all the newest stuff

3. WHAT IS YOUR FAVORITE COLOR OF LIPSTICK?

A) Red or bright pink

B) I prefer lip gloss

C) I like a light, shimmery color because it goes with everything

4. HOW LONG DO YOU SPEND ON YOUR MAKEUP DURING THE DAY?

A) No more than a minute (or however long it takes to apply lip gloss)

B) Probably 30 minutes in the morning and then a few minutes after lunch and at the end of the day

C) I'll spend about 10 minutes in the morning and then forget about it for the rest of the day

5. HOW MANY LIPSTICKS DO YOU OWN?

A) Between five and ten

B) More than 10

C) One to four

6. ONE OF THE LATEST MAKEUP TRENDS IS BRIGHTLY COLORED EYE SHADOW. HAVE YOU TRIED IT?

A) Been there, done that

B) Not my thing

C) I tried a light lavender, which looked cute

7. WHERE DO YOU BUY YOUR PRODUCTS?

A) Drugstores

B) A mix of drugstores and department stores

C) Online sites because they get all the hard-to-find stuff

8. IF YOU GO OUT AT NIGHT, WHAT'S IN YOUR MAKEUP BAG?

A) Powder, concealer, blush, lip liner, and lipstick

B) Powder and lipstick

C) Lip gloss

9. WHICH MOVIE DO YOU THINK HAD THE COOLEST MAKEUP LOOKS?

A) *Mean Girls*

B) *Wimbledon*

C) *Princess Diaries*

10. WHAT'S YOUR IDEA OF A PERFECT DATE?

A) Can you say Blockbuster?

B) Dinner for two

C) A huge party with friends

YOUR SCORE:

1. A=3 B=2 C=1	6. A=3 B=1 C=2
2. A=2 B=1 C=3	7. A= 1 B=2 C=3
3. A=3 B=1 C=2	8. A=3 B=2 C=1
4. A=1 B=3 C=2	9. A=3 B=1 C=2
5. A=2 B=3 C=1	10. A=1 B=2 C=3

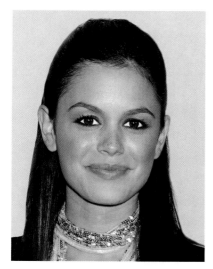

Your score . . . 10–16

Your makeup muse is: *Rachel Bilson*

Your makeup motto is . . . keep it simple.

WHY IT'S GREAT: You've got a totally mellow attitude when it comes to makeup, which is terrific. You've mastered the basics—how to cover up a zit, put on blush, and what lip color works on you. You like your face to be fairly natural looking and are a huge fan of multitasking products like those big pencils that work on both lips and cheeks, because they make your life easier. Experiment with new colors and try out some new looks. Flip to "Our All-Time Favorite Celeb Makeup Looks" on pages 64–73 for some all-star advice. And when shopping, remember that even though some colors look super bright in the package, they can be quite sheer when you try them on.

PRODUCT TO TRY: Add some sparkle to your everyday look by blending a dot of a sheer shimmer cream along the top of your cheekbones. Also, put a dot of the same shimmer cream in the middle of your bottom lip and then blend with clear gloss for a pretty pout.

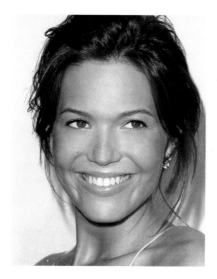

Your score . . . 17–24

You makeup muse is: *Mandy Moore*

Your makeup motto is . . . perfectly pretty.

WHY IT'S GREAT: You have no problem subtly updating your look every now and then, but you prefer classic looks: black or brown eyeliner, pink blush, and natural-looking lipstick. The trick is to make minor, yet visible, changes. Instead of buying a tomato red lipstick that all the stars are wearing, try a sheerer gloss version. Or go for a fun nail polish—toenails can handle any shade from deep plum to glittery green. Don't bother going out to buy all-new makeup; work with what you have to create a new look: mix together two lipsticks to create a different shade or use eye shadow as eyeliner by applying it with a wet cotton swab instead of the regular applicator.

PRODUCT TO TRY: A shimmery body cream. Smooth a dollop of cream onto tops of shoulders, breastbone, shins, and kneecaps for a princesslike glimmer.

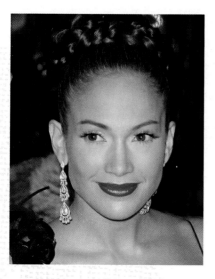

Your score . . .25–30

You makeup muse is: *Jennifer Lopez*

Your makeup motto is . . . glam slam.

WHY IT'S GREAT: You're fearless when it comes to your looks—you like to try everything, whether it's smoky green eyes or deep maroon lips (or both). When you walk into a room, everyone turns to see what head-turning look you've come up with today, and looks to you for inspiration. Just remember: if you're wearing a lot of makeup, you need to take good care of your skin and make sure you wash your face twice a day with a good cleanser (for advice on choosing a cleanser, see "What's Your Skin Type?" on page 26). Hollywood makeup artists say that great makeup always starts with good skin. If you wear a lot of eye makeup, you should also use a separate eye makeup remover since they're more gentle than the stuff you use to clean your face.

PRODUCT TO TRY: Lighten your look and even out your skin tone by trying a tinted moisturizer—look for one that also contains an SPF to protect your skin from sun damage.

YOUR TRUE COLORS

Before you put any makeup on your face, you need to figure out which shades will work best with your coloring. Just because you love Avril's smoky eyes in her new video or Hilary Duff's peachy cheeks in her new movie doesn't mean you can wear the exact same shades.

Most of the time you can wear some version of the look you love as long as the shade works with your skin tone and hair color. For example, you love bright red lips. That's great. But depending on your complexions, you and your best friend may be buying two very different "red" lipsticks to get the same look. That's because there are tons of red options out there, ranging from reds that have a lot of blue in them to reds that are packed with orange. And, depending on what color your skin and hair are, you may fall in the blue-red, orange-red, or somewhere-in-between-red. Read on to find your perfect color palette.

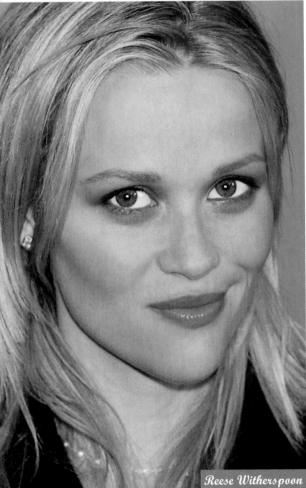

Reese Witherspoon

Fair skin and light hair

CHEEKS: Choose blush colors that mirror your natural blush. "Pale peaches and pinks will flatter your skin tone beautifully," says Mally Roncal, who pretties up the likes of Beyoncé, Alicia Keys, and Tara Reid. "Apricots and mauves are slightly more intense colors and therefore a bit more dramatic, so they are a great option for dressy evenings," adds D'Andre Michael, who makes up celebs such as Mýa and Raven.

EYES: Fair complexions can wear basically any color eye shadow, as long as it's on the lighter end of the spectrum. "Deck your lids with anything from pale green, powder blue, or light beige to lavender or pale pink," says Michael. "Keep your eyeliner pale too, by simply applying shadow as liner along your top and bottom lash lines with a thin brush, then blur the line with your finger," adds Roncal. Skip black mascara in favor of dark brown, which will look softer against your skin.

LIPS: Make your lips stand out with beautiful color. "Almost anything pastel goes," according to Valerie Sarnelle, who does makeup for Hilary Duff, Kelly Osbourne, and Sarah Jessica Parker. "Try pinks, peaches, lavenders, and soft neutrals." All these colors are great low-key choices for daytime, since they look pretty with your complexion. Bold reds and burgundies are fun to wear at night.

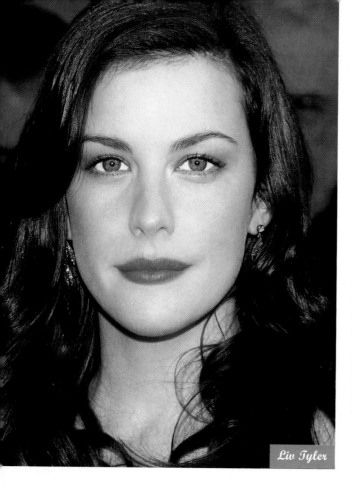

Liv Tyler

Fair skin and medium or dark hair

CHEEKS: "Add a natural-looking flush to your cheeks with medium peach, pink, and mauve shades," says Michael. Another option: if you are in the mood to create a sun-kissed glow, "go for a shimmery pale golden bronze blush," adds Roncal.

EYES: Play up your medium or dark tresses with color that's not too light and not too dark, but somewhere in between. "Try medium plum, purple, lavender, green, or blue eye shadows," recommends Roncal—they look perfect when set between the extremes of light skin and dark hair. Brown shades, across the board—"from light beige to deep chocolate"—will also look great on you, says Michael. If you want to line your eyes, use the same color shadow that you applied to your lids; an eyeliner in the same hue will also do the trick. Use black mascara to coat your upper and lower lashes.

LIPS: Shade your lips with colors that fall between light and dark, just like your eye makeup, to complement both your pale skin and dark hair. "Try reds, medium dark pinks, berries, deep corals, or pinkish browns," says Roncal.

Olive skin and medium or dark hair

CHEEKS: "Go for fun, bright colors, which stand out more against your olive complexion, like plums, red-browns, and roses," says Roncal—they will bring your face to life. "Bronzes with a bit of shimmer also look pretty, since they make you look as if you have a golden tan," adds Sarnelle.

EYES: When it comes to shadows, you've got many options. For a subtle sunny look, "browns a bit darker than your own skin and glimmery golds look great," says Roncal. Michael adds, "Bright colors—across the board—will stand against your skin and hair. Try greens, aquas, purples, or blues," he says. To really make your eyes stand out, highlight your brow bone with shimmery off-white shadow. Your eyeliner should be charcoal, black, or navy; go for jet-black mascara.

LIPS: "Make your lips stand out against your olive skin tone with red shades, like brick and wine, or more natural hues, like yummy caramels and chocolate browns," says Roncal.

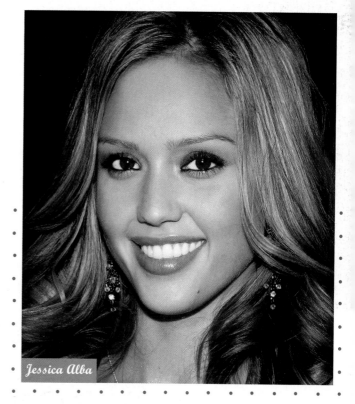

Jessica Alba

Medium golden skin and dark or medium hair

CHEEKS: "Pink, wine, and plum are your best shades to use to create a pretty flush," says Michael.

EYES: Use pale gray, slate blue, purple, or pink eye shadow on your eyelids—"these are colors that will stand out against your skin tone and brighten up your eye area," says Roncal. If you want to accent the crease, use a shadow one shade darker than the eye shadow that is on your eyelids. Highlight the brow bone with an off-white shadow. The prettiest eyeliner look for you is black or gray, since it will make the whites of your eyes look even whiter. Top off your lashes with black mascara.

LIPS: "Pink is always pretty and the most natural-looking choice for golden skin, since that's the natural color of your mouth," says Roncal. When you apply a pink shade, you're really just enhancing what is already there, plus it stands out beautifully against your skin tone. "Other colors that will look pretty with your complexion are plums, reds, and mauves," adds Michael.

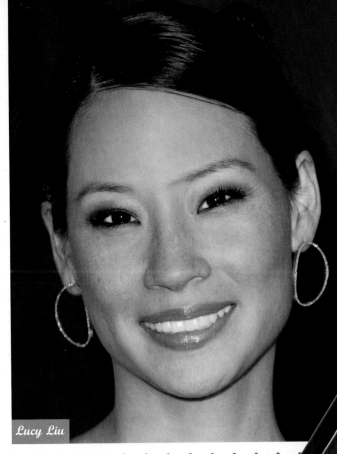

Lucy Liu

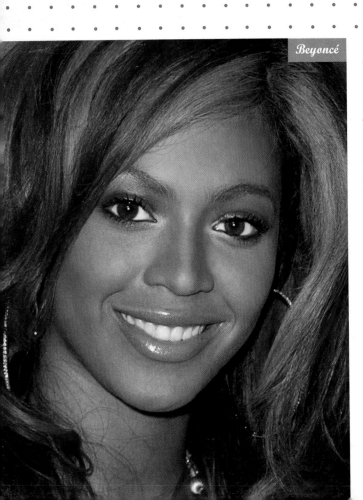

Beyoncé

Light brown skin and dark, medium, or light hair

CHEEKS: "Orange-y peach colors work really well with your skin," says Roncal. Or, "fake the look of a golden tan with bronze and gold blushes," adds Michael.

EYES: "Define your eyes in a way that looks very natural with a brown eye shadow that's infused with shimmer," suggests Sarnelle. Or have a little more fun with color by decking lids "with vibrant, sheer shades that look pretty against your light brown skin; try shimmery greens, blues, or purples," says Michael. To emphasize your brow bone, highlight it with a light brown shimmery shadow that's a few shades lighter than your natural skin tone. Deck your upper and lower lashes with black mascara.

LIPS: Add shine to your lips with glosses in natural earth tones packed with gold flecks, like light browns, caramels, brick reds, and corals," says Roncal. They will look pretty against your light brown skin.

Dark skin and dark hair

CHEEKS: For a blush to stand out and create a pretty flush against your deep skin tone, try "deep reddish shades, like rose, brick red, rust, and burgundy," says Michael. Deep mauves will make your face look fresh and are a great option for daytime looks.

EYES: To make your eyes look bright, "choose an eye shadow that's one shade lighter than your skin tone and is packed with gold or silver shiny specs," recommends Roncal. Then use an even lighter shade of eye shadow to highlight your brow bone. "For a more colorful look, coat your eyelids in deep purple or burgundy," says Michael. Line upper and lower lash lines with dark colors like gray, brown, black, or dark purple that will stand out against your skin and make your eye shape look more defined. Deck lashes in black mascara.

LIPS: Dark, juicy colors such as "deep plums, reds, rich wines, and berries make your pout stand out beautifully against your darker complexion," says Michael. "Bright colors like reds, orange, and fuchsia will look pretty for a night out," adds Sarnelle.

Brandy

HUE KNEW?

If you want to focus **ONLY** on your eyes—they are the windows to your soul, after all—and make their color look super vibrant, forget about your hair and skin coloring for a moment. (Don't forget about them forever, though. Your eyes are just one feature on your face and you can get certainly get away with putting hair color and skin tone considerations aside, occasionally.) With that in mind, we put together a palette of eye shadow shades that are guaranteed to make your eye color pop. Tip: when trying these shadow shades, keep the rest of your makeup (cheeks and lips) soft and natural, so your eyes play center stage.

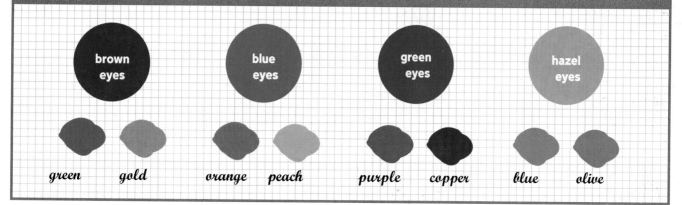

brown eyes	blue eyes	green eyes	hazel eyes
green *gold*	*orange* *peach*	*purple* *copper*	*blue* *olive*

GETTING GORGEOUS!

$\mathcal{I}$f you've already checked out the previous section, "Your True Colors," you've got a handle on which makeup shades you should be choosing. But before you go out and spend lots of money on new products, read on . . . because there's a world of choices out there!

In this section, we gathered tips from cool celebrity makeup artists Bobby Joy, Nick Barose, Jennifer Turchi, and Darrell Redleaf about the different makeup options, and how and when to use them to get totally gorgeous!

Perfect Skin

A flawless face is no longer reserved for the famous and fabulous few lucky enough to have the pros doing their makeup. Everybody—and that means you—can have perfect-looking skin, thanks to the many foundation and concealer options now available. Celebrity makeup artist Bobby Joy, who perfects the looks of stars like Lucy Liu, shares his advice about which formulation is best for which type of skin and how to put it on so it looks natural.

"It is always best to use the least amount of foundation and concealer possible, and to cover only areas that need it—not your entire face," recommends Joy. Otherwise, you can end up looking like you are wearing a mask.

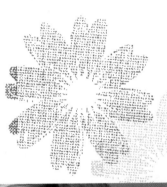

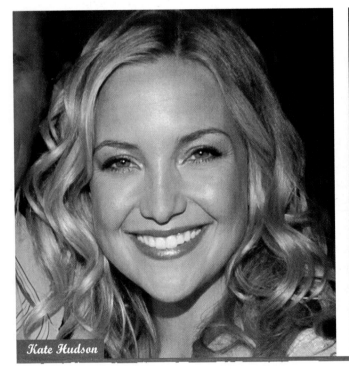

Kate Hudson

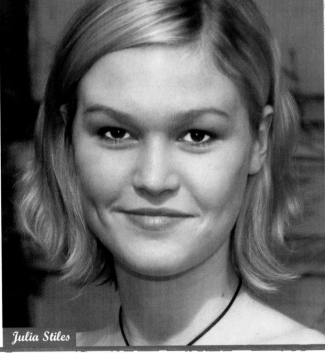

Julia Stiles

FINDING THE RIGHT FOUNDATION SHADE:

Before you figure out what kind of foundation formula you would like to try, it is important to know first what shade will work for you. Look for a shade that is the closest match possible to your skin. Then find one with "yellow" tones (think of it as a yellowish version of your own skin tone). The yellow tone will neutralize any redness in your skin, like pimples, or red splotchy areas. Foundations that have "pink" tones will only highlight redness in your skin, and you will end up looking totally unnatural.

Now that you've got that straight, here are a few shopping tips:

Drugstore

Hold a few foundations that look like they might be a close match to your skin tone up to your jaw bone. Pick the one that is the closest match. **Inside scoop:** "Most drugstore-brand foundations are made to match a range of skin tones, so an almost perfect match is likely to look great once it is blended on your face," says Joy. If you have to choose between one that is a little bit lighter or a little bit darker, go for the lighter version.

Department store

Department store brands have more shade options so you should be able to find one that matches your skin tone exactly, plus you have beauty advisors that can help you find your match, so speak up and ask for help. Dab a few options that look like close matches onto your jaw and up to your cheek. Grab a portable mirror and walk outside into the natural light to see which shade literally disappears into your skin—that's your match.

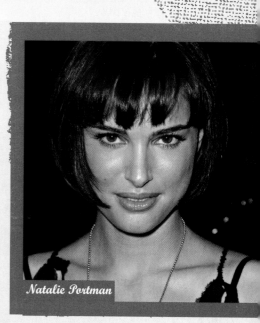

Natalie Portman

FINDING THE RIGHT FOUNDATION FORMULA:

You have a huge range of options, from see-through tints that are packed with moisture to cream to powder opaque coverage. The trick is to use the formulation that best suits your needs.

Tinted Moisturizer

TYPE OF COVERAGE: A wash of see-through color that also moisturizes your skin.

WHAT IT'S GOOD FOR: "Use a tinted moisturizer to even out your skin but still have it look natural," advises Joy.

APPLICATION TIPS: Tinted moisturizer is the easiest to apply of all the foundation options. Use your pointer and middle fingers to apply it in a thin layer. "You can always add more, so start with just a little," says Joy.

Liquid Foundation

TYPE OF COVERAGE: Sheer to medium coverage that looks dewy or matte, depending on which type you buy.

WHAT IT'S GOOD FOR: Evening out skin tone.

APPLICATION TIPS: "For even, super-thin coverage, use an angled sponge (for more info on sponges, see "Tools of the Trade" on page 54) to apply liquid foundation on flaws only—like red splotches," says Joy. Take a clean sponge and dip a corner into the liquid foundation, picking up a tiny bit of foundation. Too much foundation on the sponge will result in too much on your face and it will look heavy. Using small, quick downward strokes, dab the sponge onto the areas of your face that need coverage. Work in a downward motion, so you don't make the little hairs on your face stand on end.

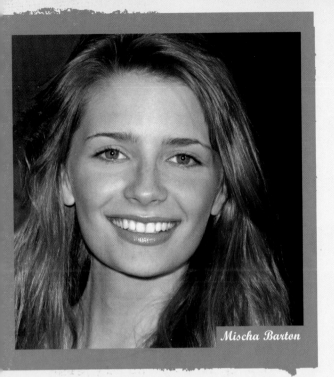

Mischa Barton

Stick Foundation

TYPE OF COVERAGE: Creamy, medium to full coverage (beautyspeak for: it's pretty darn thick).

WHAT IT'S GOOD FOR: It's great for covering up flaws, like dark circles under your eyes and redness around your nose. "It's too thick to use all over your face," according to Joy.

APPLICATION TIPS: Use it only to camouflage problem areas. "When applying, don't swipe the foundation stick directly onto your face or too much of the product will land on your skin and look unnatural," say Joy. Instead, dab the stick with a clean fingertip, then pat the foundation directly onto spots that need coverage. Don't rub or you will end up wiping it off rather than putting it on.

Cream-to-Powder Foundation

TYPE OF COVERAGE: Full coverage (beautyspeak for really, really, really thick coverage) that dries into a matte look (translation: a flat, not-shiny-at-all finish).

WHAT IT'S GOOD FOR: "Covering up flaws, like any redness on your face, but *not* for all over your face," says Joy.

APPLICATION TIP: Lightly dab the corner of a sponge into the product, picking up the tiniest amount. Then, with a light hand, work the sponge in short, downward swiping motions to apply coverage only where you need it.

Medicated Foundation

TYPE OF COVERAGE: Usually found in a liquid form, which offers creamy, medium to full coverage.

WHAT IT'S GOOD FOR: "Camouflaging and treating zits at the same time, since the foundations contain acne treatment ingredients, such as salicylic acid," says Joy.

APPLICATION TIPS: Wash your hands to clean away any dirt and bacteria (which can lead to more pimples if they come in contact with your face). Use your pointer and middle fingers to apply small amounts of foundation to problem areas on your face, like red patches. When applying the foundation, simply pat a tiny amount of foundation onto one area at a time and blend—don't rub it in or you will just wipe the product off your face.

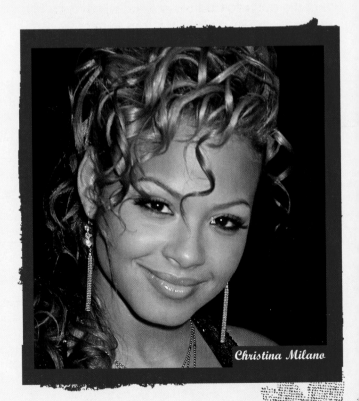

Christina Milano

PRO TIP:

Whatever type of foundation you opt for, the foundation should be oil-free, non-comedogenic (won't cause black- or whiteheads), non-acnegenic (won't cause pimples), contain sunblock of SPF 8 or higher, and be hypoallergenic (won't cause allergic reactions).

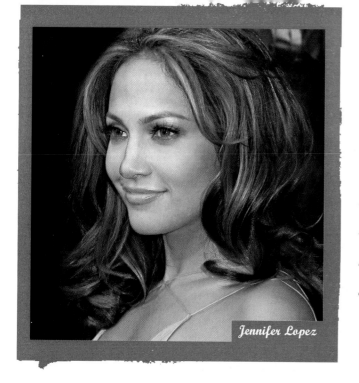

Jennifer Lopez

Concealer

TYPE OF COVERAGE: Concealers are creams that are even heavier than foundations and are usually found in little pots, sticks, and tubes.

WHAT IT'S GOOD FOR: Use concealers sparingly on spots that need extra help, like under your eyes to cover dark circles. When choosing a concealer color use the same method we talked about in "Finding the Right Foundation Shade."

APPLICATION TIPS: Concealers go on way too thickly if you apply them directly from a stick or wand. Instead, dab a tad on the back of your hand, rub it with your index finger to warm it up and thin it out (so it looks natural on your skin), then dot it on the problem zone. Wait three seconds, and blend it out with a clean finger. "To keep your concealer in place, after it has dried, top it with loose translucent powder applied with a powder brush," says Joy.

Translucent Loose Powder

WHAT IT IS: Powder loosely contained in a jar—as opposed to hard pressed, such as powder eye shadow or blush. While it can look like it is an off-white color in the jar, when applied, it blends into your skin color.

WHAT IT'S GOOD FOR: Dusting over your makeup to create a thin film that will keep your makeup in place longer, absorbing oil and stopping shine.

APPLICATION TIPS: Tap a big fluffy powder brush into the powder, so the bristles pick up a very small amount. Then, tap the handle of the brush against your palm to remove even more powder—you don't want to apply too much and end up looking like a dust bunny! With loose powder, less is definitely more. Lightly brush the remaining powder onto areas of your face where you have applied foundation, like over your pimples.

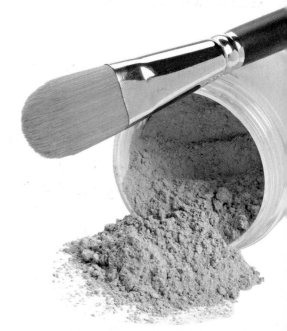

BEAUTIFUL EYES

Want high-profile peepers? The first step to starry eyes is to understand eye makeup products and what they are good for. After you've got this section down, you can flip to "All Eyes on Hollywood" on page 56 for specific how-tos, tips, and tricks on eye makeup looks that suit every eye shape and size. Here, Hollywood makeup artist Nick Barose, who works on celebs like Scarlett Johansson and Michelle Branch, gives you a behind-the-scenes look at all your eye makeup options, from shadows to pencils and mascaras.

EYE SHADOW 101

POWDER EYE SHADOW

WHAT IT IS: Eye color that is in the form of a pressed powder, which is available in everything from pale to bold hues and tons of finishes, including matte, shimmery, and glittery. The coverage can be anywhere from sheer (for a subtle tint), to almost opaque (so you can barely see through it).

WHAT IT'S GOOD FOR: "It is ideal for creating dressy eye makeup looks, since you can layer two to three colors onto your lids—one shade on your eyelid, one shade in the crease, and one shade on the brow bone," says Barose.

CREAM EYE SHADOW

WHAT IT IS: A cream color for eyes that comes in either a stick, pot, or tube.

WHAT IT'S GOOD FOR: According to Barose, "It's a quick and easy way to cover lids with a single see-through color, which looks fun and fresh." Also available are cream-to-powder shadows, which are like their cream sisters, but offer bolder, less see-through coverage. But be warned: Both types of cream eye shadows can settle into the tiny creases on your lids and can end up looking messy, so don't forget to touch up the look by wiping away the old crease-y shadow and apply a fresh coat.

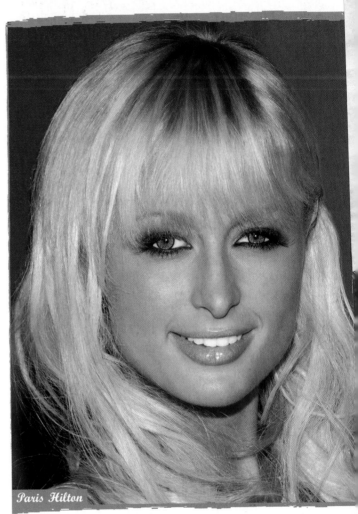

Paris Hilton

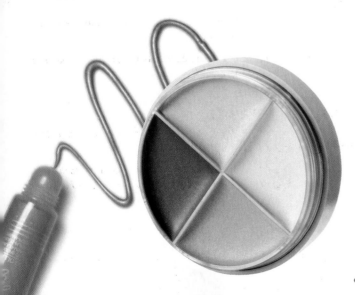

EYE GLOSS

WHAT IT IS: A very shiny see-through eye color, which is like a lip gloss for your eyelids.

WHAT IT'S GOOD FOR: "This type of shadow will really make your lids stand out since the color is so bright and shiny," says Barose. But the color may sink into your little eye creases, like the cream shadows, so touch up throughout the day by wiping away the old crease-y shadow and apply a fresh coat.

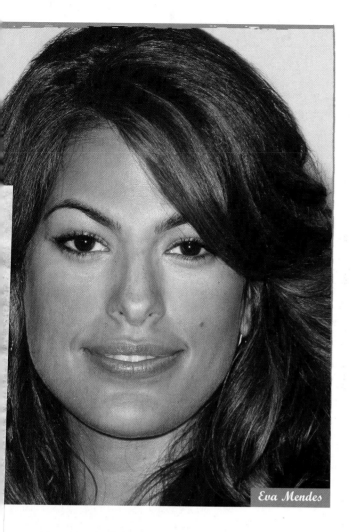

Eva Mendes

EYELINER 101

EYELINER PENCIL

WHAT IT IS: A wax-based pencil used to line the eyes.

WHAT IT'S GOOD FOR: It creates soft lines along your upper and lower lash lines.

LIQUID EYELINER

WHAT IT IS: Either a felt-tipped pen or tiny brush covered with liquid. If you are just learning, the pens are easier to use than the liquid/brush combos.

WHAT IT'S GOOD FOR: Creating a dramatic look with a perfectly neat line—that is, not smudged like an eye pencil—on your upper and lower lash lines.

MASCARA 101

CURLING MASCARA

WHAT IT IS: A mascara that has a formula that makes lashes curl and look darker, or a wand with curved, uneven bristles to add color and curl to your lashes. Either way, lashes come out looking flirty!

WHAT IT'S GOOD FOR: "Making your eyes look wide open, since lashes curl up, up, and away," says Barose.

THICKENING MASCARA

WHAT IT IS: A mascara in which the formula is made to pump up each lash. Also, the mascara wand has bristles spaced far apart and therefore has room to hold lots of that lash-thickening formula, which goes on super thick.

WHAT IT'S GOOD FOR: "Making a statement, since your lashes will look so thick," says Barose.

LENGTHENING MASCARA

WHAT IT IS: "A mascara with a wand with bristles that are flexible and very close together, so it can grip your lashes and add mascara formula all the way from the lash base to just beyond the natural tips of your lashes," says Barose.

WHAT IT'S GOOD FOR: Creating a delicate eyelash look, since this mascara adds length to your lashes without making them look thicker.

LASH TINT

WHAT IT IS: A mascara that only adds color, not length or width (a.k.a. thickness), to your lashes.

WHAT IT'S GOOD FOR: "Lash tints are great for making your lashes stand out a little bit more than they normally do with color, while keeping the look very natural, since there is no added length or thickness," explains Barose.

CLEAR MASCARA

WHAT IT IS: A mascara that has no color, but instead makes lashes stand out softly with a clear finish.

WHAT IT'S GOOD FOR: Making your lashes look shiny yet natural as there is no added color, thickness, or length.

WATERPROOF MASCARA

WHAT IT IS: A mascara that will not come off when you are underwater, sweating, or tearing up.

WHAT IT'S GOOD FOR: Dressing up your eyes for a trip to the beach, pool, or prom, because it won't run down your face when wet.

CHEEK IT OUT!

Sure, an Oscar or a Grammy award can put a glow in any star's cheeks—just look at Beyoncé's and Gwen Stefani's—but so can a bit of blush. Jennifer Turchi, who blushes up Lucy Liu and Christina Ricci on a regular basis, gives you goof-proof guidance on getting a glam glow.

Powder Blush

WHAT IT IS: Powder blush makes the boldest statement because coverage tends to be medium to heavy. It's best on normal, combination, and oily skin.

WHAT IT'S GOOD FOR: Use it to create a healthy-looking flush when applied to cheek apples as well as to contour cheekbones, since you can be precise with a makeup brush.

PREP COURSE: If your skin feels dry, apply an oil-free moisturizer with SPF 15 all over your face after cleansing to make your skin smooth enough for powder to go on evenly, without streaks. Wait a couple of minutes for the moisturizer to sink in before applying blush.

APPLICATION TIP: "Grab a dome-shaped blush brush, not a fat bronzer brush or a fluffy powder brush (for more info on brushes, see "Tools of the Trade" on page 54), but the perfectly in-between blush brush," says Turchi. Swab the brush over the blush in a circle. "Smile at the mirror, and use short, delicate strokes to sweep blush onto the apples of your cheek (the part that sticks out when you smile) and up toward your temple," she explains. Blend so the blush looks natural—no lines or streaks allowed!

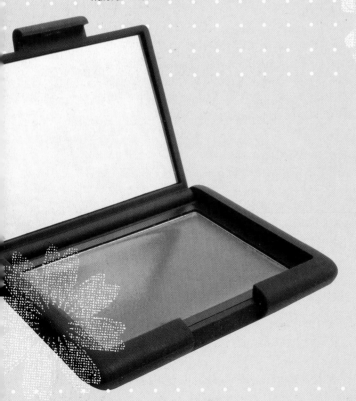

Cream Blush

WHAT IT IS: Cream blush offers plenty of color, but it's sheer enough to let skin show through; "it literally looks like the color is shining from underneath your skin," says Turchi.

WHAT IT'S GOOD FOR: It's softer and less dramatic than powder blush, and its creamy texture means it's best for normal to dry skin.

PREP COURSE: If your skin feels dry, apply an oil-free moisturizer with SPF 15 all over your face to get it blush ready. Wait a couple of minutes for it to absorb before applying blush.

APPLICATION TIP: "Smile and use your index finger to gently tap three small dots onto the apples of your cheeks (the part that sticks out when you smile), then use small circular motions to blend color up and out," recommends Turchi.

Liquid Blush

WHAT IT IS: A liquid blush gives you a finish that is more matte than other types of blush.

WHAT IT'S GOOD FOR: Liquids "stain" your cheeks, so the sheer color stays put for hours. They look best on oily, combination, and normal skin types.

PREP COURSE: Smooth, well-moisturized skin is essential because a liquid needs to glide on easily—"so apply right after you moisturize your face" if you have dry skin, says Turchi.

APPLICATION TIP: A liquid stains your face in a snap, so the trick is to get it on right the first time. Most liquids come as a roll-on for easier application. Apply blots of color to the center of your cheek apples, then quickly blend the color with your finger—in large circular motions—over and just beyond the apples of your cheeks (the part that sticks out when you smile).

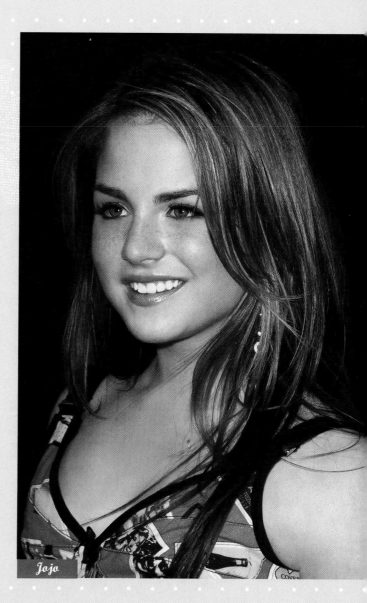

Jojo

Gel Blush

WHAT IT IS: "Gels offer the sheerest, freshest color," says Turchi—you can even use them on other areas besides your cheeks, like your lips.

WHAT IT'S GOOD FOR: The magic of gels is that they're so light, they make you look like you just got a surprise kiss from your crush. They're great on oily and combo types, but are not so good on dry skin—if you have any flakiness or cracks, this blush can make them stand out.

PREP COURSE: Smooth skin is key, so apply after exfoliating with a mild scrub to even out surface texture. Then, if your skin feels dry, apply an oil-free moisturizer with SPF 15 and let it set for a few minutes.

APPLICATION TIP: To create a breathlessly fresh face, dab your finger in moisturizer, then top with a tiny bit of gel blush, mix together, and apply to the center of your cheeks and blend up and out toward your temples.

LIP SERVICE

From air kisses on the red carpet to smooches with a hot leading man on screen, where would stars be without a perfect pout? One of the best things about making up your lips is having so many formulas to choose from. Makeup pro Darrell Redleaf, who plays up the puckers of stars like Scarlett Johansson, Cameron Diaz, and Joss Stone, tells you all about your lipstick options.

LIPSTICK 101

LIP GLOSS

WHAT IT IS: A sheer, wet-looking formula that can range from clear to colorful.

WHAT IT'S GOOD FOR: Creating a thin coat of color that looks subtle, since your natural lip color shows through. Glosses are a surefire way to pretty up your pout instantly—day or night.

APPLICATION TIPS: "Use your fingertip, a brush, or sponge-tipped applicator to apply gloss to the center of your mouth, on both your upper and lower lips," recommends Redleaf. Then smush your lips together and move them back and forth to distribute color.

CREAM LIPSTICK

WHAT IT IS: A creamy formula that is packed with rich color, so it offers medium to full coverage. The color falls somewhere between flat and shiny.

WHAT IT'S GOOD FOR: Making lips stand out with opaque color, plus adding moisture to lips at the same time. Cream lipsticks are great for special occasions or at night, since they can make your lips stand out in the dimmest of light.

APPLICATION TIP: Since cream lipsticks stand out more than glosses, precise, neat application is key. If the point of your lipstick has been rounded off from tons of use, "use a lip brush (read all about them in "Tools of the Trade" on page 54) to apply lipstick by dabbing it on your lipstick, then painting lipstick directly on lips," says Redleaf. Whether you are applying color directly from the lipstick tube or using a brush, start at the center of the top lip and work outward, one side at a time. Do the same to your lower lip.

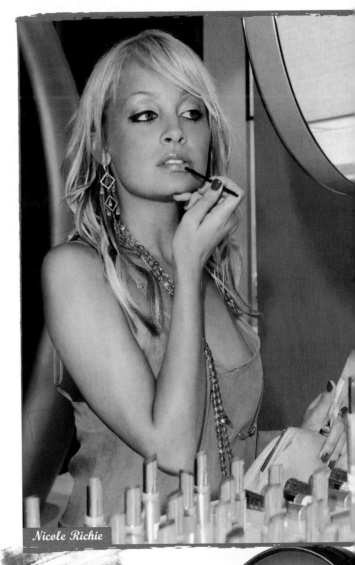

Nicole Richie

CELEB SECRET TIP: Since all eyes will be on your lips, make them as smooth as possible. Coat your mouth with tons of lip balm, then work an old soft toothbrush over your lips in a back and forth motion to remove flaky dead skin. Keep your mouth in tip-top shape by applying lip balm every night before bed.

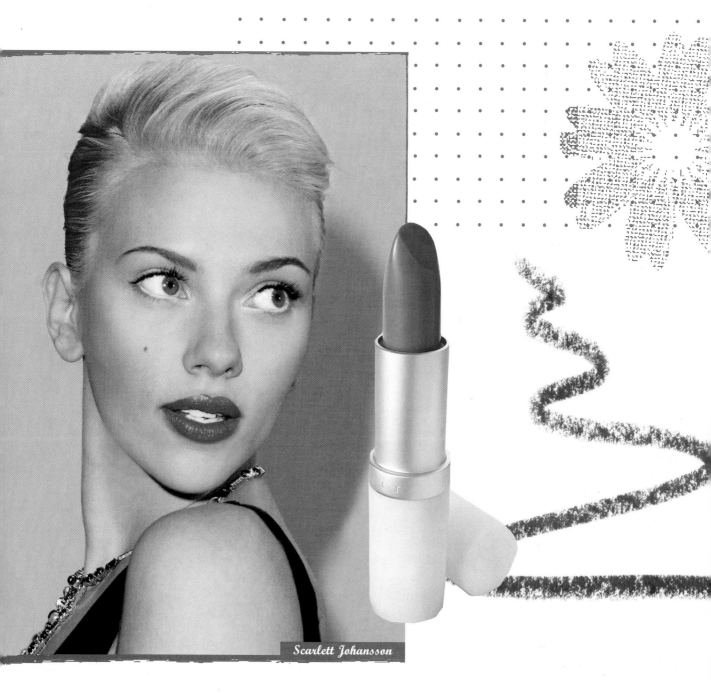

Scarlett Johansson

MATTE LIPSTICK

WHAT IT IS: Intense, opaque color that has no sheen or shimmer (basically, matte means flat).

WHAT IT'S GOOD FOR: Since this lipstick option can look a bit severe, it is best kept for creating a dramatic look for a night out on the town. Think prom.

APPLICATION TIP: "Matte lipstick can be drying, so before applying, treat lips to a moisturizing lip balm," says Redleaf. Next, apply the lipstick carefully with a lip brush (for more makeup brush info, see "Tools of the Trade" on page 54), since matte lipstick is an attention grabber.

LIP LINER

WHAT IT IS: A pencil that is packed with lip color.

WHAT IT'S GOOD FOR: Use it to define the shape of your lips, stop lipstick from bleeding (a.k.a. going out of the lines), and help lipstick last longer.

APPLICATION TIP: To create a precise line right at the edge of your lips, start at the center of your top lip (called the bow) and draw a line to the outer right corner. Go back to the center and draw a line to the outer left corner. Do the same on your bottom lip.

TOOLS OF THE TRADE

To apply makeup properly and glam yourself up like the stars, the right tools are essential. Once you've seen what a blush brush can do or the life-saving precision of a super-pointy lip brush, you will never use anything else. But a girl could be forgiven if she looked at a handful of brushes and other assorted items and couldn't figure out which ones were best to use with what—that's where we come in. The following is the 411 on everything you need, from brushes to tweezers, to make yourself up like a pro.

BRUSHES

LIP BRUSH

WHAT IT IS: A short, stiff-bristled brush that's used for lipstick or gloss. Retractable versions are great for dumping in your purse.

WHAT TO DO WITH IT: Cover the bristles in your fave lip shade by dipping the brush into a pot of gloss or rubbing it over the top of a lipstick and paint in your lips for a precise application.

TIP: To guarantee a perfect lip line, make a half grin to stretch out the skin while you fill in.

EYE SHADOW BRUSH

WHAT IT IS: A small brush with fluffy bristles that's used to sweep shadows over your lids. Bristle shapes vary from rounded to flat at the tips—the rounded versions are the easiest to use.

WHAT TO DO WITH IT: Use it to apply powder eye shadows on your lids from lash line to crease or sweep it through your crease for a more dramatic look.

TIP: You can also use this brush to highlight your brow bone (with a powder shadow that's a shade lighter than your skin tone).

BROW BRUSH

WHAT IT IS: A stiff-bristled brush used to neaten the look of brows.

WHAT TO DO WITH IT: Brush unruly eyebrows into place by working brow hairs up and out toward your temples.

TIP: To keep brows in place, slick a little clear lip gloss over your brows, then brush it through.

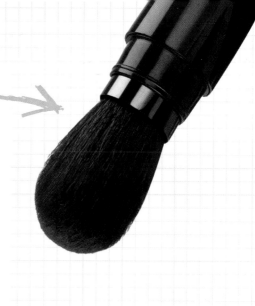

BLUSH BRUSH

WHAT IT IS: A medium-size brush with bristles that angle down to one side.

WHAT TO DO WITH IT: Since blush can look fake if you overload the brush, start with just a little on your brush and apply more if needed. To figure out where it goes, smile in the mirror and swirl the blush on the apples (the part of your cheek that sticks out).

TIP: If you go overboard with your blush, take it down a notch with a dusting of translucent face powder.

BRONZER BRUSH

WHAT IT IS: A medium-size fluffy brush that usually has straight-edged bristles and is used to create a tan glow.

WHAT TO DO WITH IT: Since bronzers are sheer, they can be applied to multiple areas. Dip brush into product and apply everywhere the sun would naturally hit your face—like your forehead, tip of nose, chin, and cheeks. Use quick, back-and-forth motions for a natural look.

TIP: Bronzer looks great when brushed across your collarbone, especially when sporting a tank, tube, or halter top.

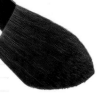

POWDER BRUSH

WHAT IT IS: The biggest and fluffiest of all brushes, which works to eliminate shine and minimize the look of your pore size.

WHAT TO DO WITH IT: To use with loose powder, dip brush tip into a container of powder and then tap it against your hand to shake off excess. For pressed powder, swirl brush in compact using a circular motion. For both, dust face starting with your greasier parts (forehead, nose, and chin) before hitting drier areas like cheeks.

TIP: Dip powder brushes into pots of shimmer or glitter, then dust over your collarbones and legs for pretty skin from head to toe.

CONCEALER BRUSH

WHAT IT IS: A small brush with slightly tapered or flat-headed bristles used to camouflage pimples.

WHAT TO DO WITH IT: Lightly dab the bristles into your cream concealer or liquid foundation, then apply the makeup to the center of a pimple. Blend color outward until it disappears into your skin.

TIP: To keep your cover-up in place, lightly dust over it with a powder brush and translucent loose powder.

MORE TOOLS

TWEEZERS

WHAT IT IS: A tool that has an angled tip that ends in a point. Used to pluck unwanted hairs.

WHAT TO DO WITH IT: Carefully tweeze one brow hair at a time, in the direction hair grows, to neaten the look of your arches.

TIP: It's less painful to tweeze brows after taking a shower, since the warm water opens up your pores.

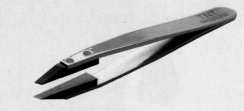

SMALL WEDGE SPONGES

WHAT IT IS: A wedge of sponge that helps you apply liquid foundation evenly.

WHAT TO DO WITH IT: Dot foundation on cheeks, chin, and forehead. Use sponge to spread color in a downward direction to keep tiny face hairs from sticking up.

TIP: Throw sponges away after a few uses, since they can trap bacteria and ultimately cause pimples.

ALL EYES ON HOLLYWOOD

*Y*ou can tell a lot about a person just by looking in her eyes. You can also tell a lot about a person by looking at her eye makeup! We rounded up the best looks for all different types of eyes as well as Tinseltown tips about what to do to really make your own peepers pop.

What's your eye shape and type?

When it comes to makeup choices for your eyes, there really are endless possibilities—for example, to line or not to line, to smudge or to smear your eyeliner and whether to try black or purple eye shadow. However, there are some basics that everyone needs to know, especially when it comes to making up different eye shapes. "Eye makeup is amazing because you can really change the shape of the eyes or make them look bigger, smaller, whatever you want," says makeup artist Agostina for Cloutier. "Because of all the products and brushes, eye makeup may seem a little tricky at first, but once you get the basics down, it's easy, and that's when you can get creative."

SMALL EYES

If your eyes seem to disappear when you apply a lot of eyeliner, chances are they're a little on the small side. These eyes are often cute and sparkly, but you'll notice that if you a see a picture of yourself smiling really wide, smaller eyes tend to almost disappear. Often, this eye shape doesn't have a large eyelid, so it's key to go easy on the makeup. The main rule is to stick to the lighter shades, since dark colors can make them appear even tinier. "The biggest mistake people with small eyes make is lining around the whole eye" says celebrity makeup artist Bruce Grayson, who has worked with Jennifer Aniston and Drew Barrymore. "A dark circle around the eye only creates a smaller-looking circle."

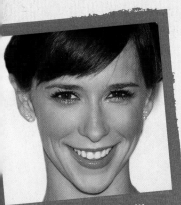

Jennifer Love Hewitt

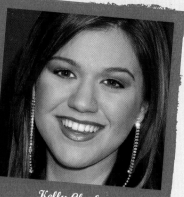

Kelly Clarkson

Do

• **CHOOSE AN EYELINER PENCIL IN A LIGHTER SHADE**, like taupe or light gray, because those colors are more subtle. Line the outer third of the top eyelid and the outer third of the bottom eyelid only. Blend with a cotton swab or freshly-washed finger to soften the look.

• **GET A WHITE EYELINER PENCIL** and line the lower inner lid (right above the lower lashes). This also makes eyes look bigger.

• **USE A PALE SHIMMERY SHADE** on the lids (anything from cream for lighter skin to bronze for darker coloring) to make eyes really stand out. Sweep color on lids up to the crease, and with whatever is left on the brush, dust color at the inner corner of the eye. Blend this shadow outward so that some of the color goes on the top lid and some goes on the bottom lid.

Don't

• **USE EYE SHADOWS IN DARK SHADES** such as black, dark navy, and chocolate brown because darker colors make eyes look even smaller.

• **SKIP THE EYELASH CURLER.** Always curl your lashes (this really opens up the eye), and apply mascara to top and bottom lashes. Here's how to curl your eyelashes: Grab the curler and hold it like a pair of scissors (using your thumb and index finger). Looking straight ahead, place the curler so that your lashes sit between the two curling pads. Clamp the curler down on lashes, count to ten, and let go. When you're done, apply a second coat of mascara.

LARGE EYES

If you look at your face in the mirror and your eyes seem to be the most prominent feature, chances are they're on the large side. Bigger eyes show a lot of eyelid and don't need as much makeup to accentuate the natural shape. While it's actually a huge asset to have large eyes because they allow for lots of choices, there are still of couple of things to keep in mind. "Larger-eyed girls should apply really simple eye makeup, without too much shading or too many contrasting colors, so that the eyes don't overpower the rest of the face," suggests Hollywood makeup artist Valerie Sarnelle, whose client list includes Kelly Osbourne, Sarah Jessica Parker, and Halle Berry.

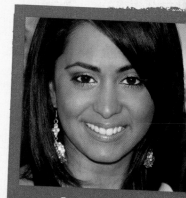

Parminder Nagra

Do

• PICK NON-SHIMMERY COLORS like khaki, dark plum, or burgundy, which work with every eye color. Place the shadow in the middle of the eyelid and blend it outward first, then inward. Stop right where the crease of your eyelid starts.

• LINE AROUND THE WHOLE EYE with a pencil (pick a dark and dramatic shade like black, navy, or gray). Larger eyes can handle a lot of eyeliner.

• MINIMIZE LARGE EYES by lining the inner rim of the lower eyelid (above the eyelashes) with the same dark eye pencil that you used on the top eyelid.

Don't

• WEAR TOO MANY DIFFERENT EYE SHADOW SHADES on the lid all at once. Since a lot of your eyelid is exposed, three or four eye shadow shades at the same time will just look clownish. The easiest way is one shadow and a liner.

• PUT MASCARA ON LOWER LASHES. Coating all of your lashes can give large eyes a doll-like effect. Coloring the top lashes only gives the eyes a glam look without making them look too big.

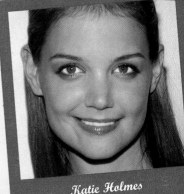

Katie Holmes

CLOSE-SET EYES

When eyes are situated fairly close together, they can make your face look smaller, because all of your features will appear to be sitting in the middle of your face (if you look at the pic of Alicia Silverstone you'll notice that her eyes, nose, and mouth are all close together). "However, it's easy to give the illusion of more widely-set eyes by concentrating most of your eye makeup on the outer corners, creating a larger, more balanced shape," says Agostina.

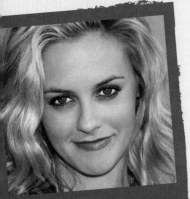

Alicia Silverstone

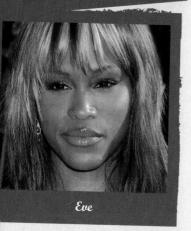

Eve

Do

• GET EYE SHADOW-APPLICATION SMART. Start with a shimmery or flat color in a light shade (creams work well for those with lighter skin tones and golds are great for darker skin tones). Brush the shadow onto the lid by placing the color right above your top eyelashes and then blending it upwards to the eyebrows. Next, take a powder eye shadow that's a few shades darker than your original shade and apply a dot on the outer third of the top eyelid. Blend it upward and out using your fingers.

• APPLY A DOT OF LIGHT SHADOW (white for lighter skin tones and light gold for darker skin tones) right at the inner corner of the eye, next to the nose (this works if you're not wearing any other eye shadow). Blend it out over the upper and lower eyelid. The light shade makes the eyes look farther apart.

Don't

• APPLY EYELINER ALL ALONG THE TOP LASH LINE. Start from the middle of the top eyelid and line outward. Also steer clear of using liner on the inner half of the eye, closest to the nose. Do the same with the lower lid. Blend the liner with a cotton swab or a freshly-washed finger to soften the look.

• APPLY MASCARA TO ALL LASHES. Color just the outer half to give the illusion of your eyes being farther apart.

DEEP-SET OR HOODED EYES

The easiest way to see if your eyes fall into this category is to look at your eyes in the mirror. If your eyelids don't have a visible crease, these tips are for you. The wrong type of makeup can make this type of eye appear smaller, but the right eye makeup can give you a very dramatic look. "This is very common for some Asian eyes, but also for other shapes," says Grayson. "The main thing to remember when applying eye makeup is go easy—a little goes a long way with this eye shape."

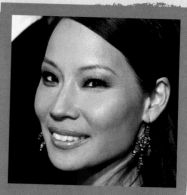

Lucy Liu

Do

• TRY EYELINER JUST ON TOP OF THE UPPER LASH LINE. Use whatever color you want, but make sure it's a darkish shade (chocolate brown, navy, plum, or black).

• MAKE YOUR EYES POP. Use a light sparkly eye shadow on the brow bone. A shimmery cream color looks great with lighter skin tones; light golds or bronzes work beautifully on darker skin tones.

Don't

• USE DARK SHADOWS ON THE LIDS. They won't really be visible on your eyes.

• SKIP MASCARA, because long lashes really open up this eye shape. For added drama, why not try a curling mascara?

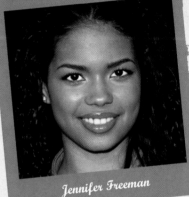

Jennifer Freeman

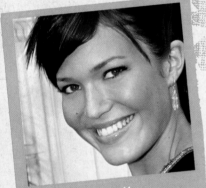

Mandy Moore

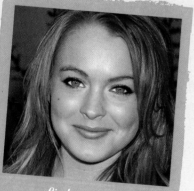

Lindsay Lohan

ALMOND EYES

Almond eyes are large, long, and often turn up a little at the outer corners. "This is the easiest type of eye to apply eye makeup to, since it is usually an average size and the slight angling is always flattering," says Agostina. Also, this eye shape usually shows just enough of the upper eyelid when the eye is open and looking forward that both liner and colored shadows will look super pretty without being overpowering. "The basic rules still apply," add Agostina, "It doesn't mean you should pile on tons of eye makeup. Almond-eyed girls just have a few more options."

Do

• APPLY ONE COAT OF MASCARA ON THE TOP LASHES. This gives it a real "cat's eye" look that is super stylish.

• APPLY A DOT OF SHIMMERY SHADOW in a neutral shade right on the brow bone (the outer half of your eyebrow). Blend the shadow outward until it disappears into the skin. This hint of glimmer creates a perfect highlight for the eyes without looking like you put on a ton of makeup.

Don't

• WEAR DARK SHADOW AND DARK LINER AT THE SAME TIME. Pick one or the other to avoid a heavy look.

• LINE AROUND YOUR WHOLE EYE. While your eyes are a good size, too much liner will make them shrink. If you love to line the lower and the upper eye, start a third of the way in from the corner closest to your nose.

OUR TOP THREE EYE LOOKS

*N*ow that you've learned what works best with your eye shape, check out these cool makeup looks. Don't be afraid to experiment with a style you've never worn before, because eye makeup is all about having fun—and hey, it's a snap to remove (with eye makeup remover of course!).

1. Lots of Liner

Why We Love It

It's seriously cool with a little punky twist. "The key to creating this type of lined eye is to keep the rest of the face very natural," says Sarnelle. "You don't need a lot of makeup on the rest of your face."

What You'll Need
- ❏ EYE SHADOW BRUSH
- ❏ COTTON SWABS
- ❏ LIGHT GRAY EYE SHADOW
- ❏ BLACK EYELINER
- ❏ BLACK MASCARA

How To Get The Look

1. Start by applying a dab of the eye shadow in the lower middle of the upper eyelid. Blend it upward and outward so that the color can just be seen above the natural crease of the eye.

2. Use black eyeliner to line the outer two-thirds of the top lash, then do a very thin line along the whole lower lash line.

3. Take a cotton swab, put a smudge of the eye shadow on the end of it, and apply it at the lower corner of the inner eye and then blend it up and over to the inner corner of the top lid.

4. Finish with a coat of black mascara on your top lashes and you're done.

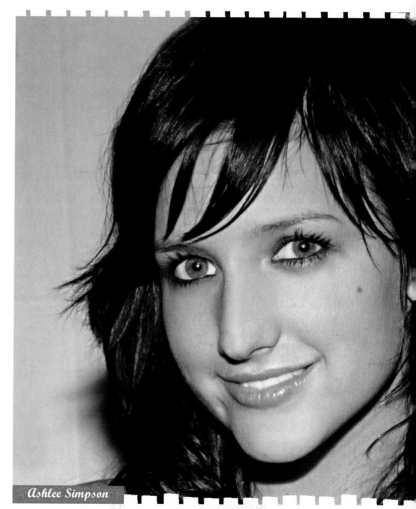

Ashlee Simpson

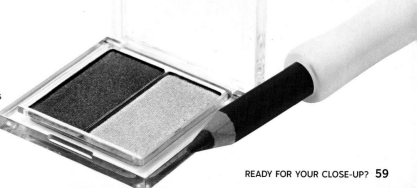

2. Smoky & Sexy

Why We Love It

It's a glam-looking lined eye with a twist. "With an eye look this strong, keep it really modern by only using neutral colors like grays and browns," suggests Grayson.

What You'll Need

- ❏ EYE SHADOW BRUSH
- ❏ COTTON SWABS
- ❏ NEUTRAL-TONED EYE SHADOW
- ❏ TAUPE EYE SHADOW
- ❏ DARK BROWN EYE SHADOW
- ❏ DARK BROWN EYELINER
- ❏ BLACK MASCARA

How To Get The Look

1. Start by dusting the whole top lid with a neutral-toned shadow—one that is your natural skin tone but just a touch brighter (in this picture Avril wears a light peachy pink).

2. Take the taupe shadow and apply a bit of it in the middle of the upper eyelid. Blend it up and outward so you can see the color just above the crease and at the outer corners.

3. Take a cotton swab and draw a line of the eye shadow all along the lower lash line, blending it a little bit along the way so there are no harsh lines.

4. Use a cotton swab to smudge a line of the dark brown shadow on the outer third of the top eyelid.

5. Line the lower eyelid with dark brown eyeliner. Smudge the line with a clean cotton swab.

6. Apply one coat of mascara to top and bottom lashes.

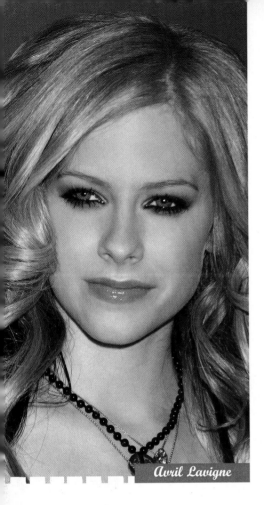

Avril Lavigne

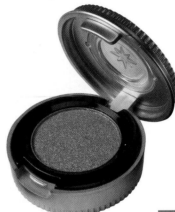

3. Color Crazy

Why We Love It

It's totally fun, and you can change your shadow as often as you change you outfit. "This is a great look," says Sarnelle. "Just keep the rest of your face neutral. Avoid wearing bright eyes with bright lips."

What You'll Need

- ❏ EYE SHADOW BRUSH
- ❏ COTTON SWABS
- ❏ LIGHT YELLOW SHIMMERY EYE SHADOW
- ❏ EMERALD GREEN SHIMMERY EYE SHADOW
- ❏ BEIGE SHIMMERY EYE SHADOW
- ❏ BLACK MASCARA

How To Get The Look

1. Start by applying the light yellow eye shadow all over the top eyelid and then blending the color up and out towards the eyebrow.

2. With a cotton swab, draw a line of green eye shadow along the top lash line from the inner corner and all the way out, winging the line upward a bit at the outer edge. Smudge color with a clean cotton swab to soften the look. Dust another smudgy line using the green eye shadow along the outer third of the lower lash line.

3. Put a dot of the beige shadow at the inner corner of the lower eyelid and blend it outward with a clean cotton swab until this color meets up with the green eye shadow.

4. Apply two coats of black mascara to the top lashes.

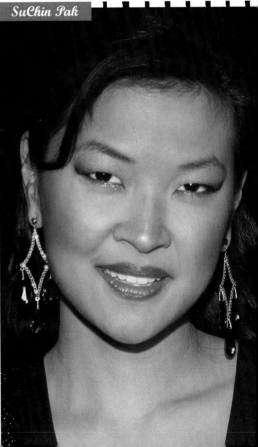

SuChin Pak

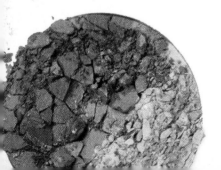

LUSCIOUS LIPS

*E*ver notice how celebs can change their entire look with the swish of a lipstick? We've seen Gwyneth Paltrow go from sweet to sultry simply by trading in petal pink gloss for a red hot cream lipstick. Lip color is one of the easiest and quickest ways to play up your mood, whether it's flirty, dramatic, or ultracool. Now that you know all about your lipstick options and how they work from "Getting Gorgeous" on page 52, it's time to try some lip looks on for size. Here are three starworthy options for you to try, with tips from celebrity makeup artist Darrell Redleaf, who plays up the puckers of stars like Scarlett Johansson and Cameron Diaz.

1. Pastel Gloss

THE LOOK: Sparkling sheer pink lips, like Paris Hilton's, are a surefire way to pretty up your look, no matter your coloring.

WHAT IT'S GOOD FOR: Gloss is so simple and versatile, you can wear it anytime—from school to date—and you are sure to look flirty.

What You'll Need
- ❏ LIP PENCIL THAT MATCHES YOUR LIP COLOR
- ❏ SHEER PALE PINK LIP GLOSS

How To Get The Look:

1. "Define lips and keep gloss from bleeding (edging out onto the skin around your mouth) by lining them with a lip pencil that matches your natural lip color," says Redleaf. Use your middle finger to blend the color inward so there are no visible lines.

2. "Apply a dollop of gloss with your fingertip, a brush, or a sponge-tipped wand to the center portion of your mouth," recommends Redleaf; gently press your lips together and smush back and forth to distribute color. Now add a bit more gloss to the outer edges.

3. Make your pout shine even more with a touch of shimmery gloss right in the center of your top and bottom lip.

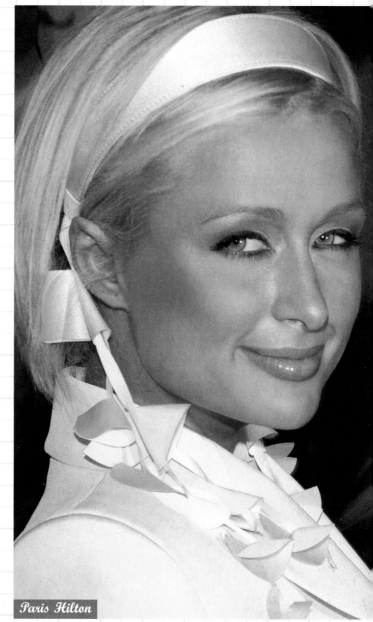

Paris Hilton

2. Red Hot

THE LOOK: Creamy red lips, like Gabrielle Union's, are chart-toppers. When people look at you, they will stop in their tracks and check out your pout.

WHAT IT'S GOOD FOR: Paint your kisser red when you want to make a statement without saying a word. Special nights, like dates and dances, are a good time to try out this daring look.

What You'll Need
- ❏ CREAMY RED LIPSTICK
- ❏ RED LIP LINER THAT MATCHES YOUR LIPSTICK
- ❏ LIP BRUSH
- ❏ TISSUES
- ❏ TRANSLUCENT POWDER
- ❏ POWDER BRUSH

How To Get The Look

1. Since red cream lipsticks can be attention grabbers, they've got to look perfectly neat. "Using a red lip liner that matches your lipstick of choice, very carefully line your lips following their natural shape, just inside your natural lip line," says Redleaf. You don't want a ring around the lips. Using the same pencil, fill in your lips.

2. For extra precision, use a little lip brush (read all about them in "Tools of the Trade" on page 54) to apply lipstick, says Redleaf. Because the brush will form a nice point, you'll have total control over where you place the color. Take the brush, pick up a bit of color from your lipstick, and apply it your lips.

3. Blot lips with tissue, or "dust over your pout with a translucent loose powder and a powder brush," says Redleaf (for more info on brushes, see "Tools of the Trade" on page 54).

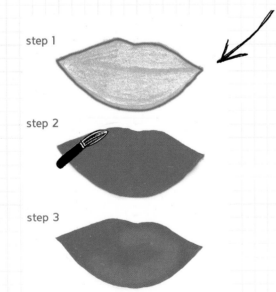

step 1

step 2

step 3

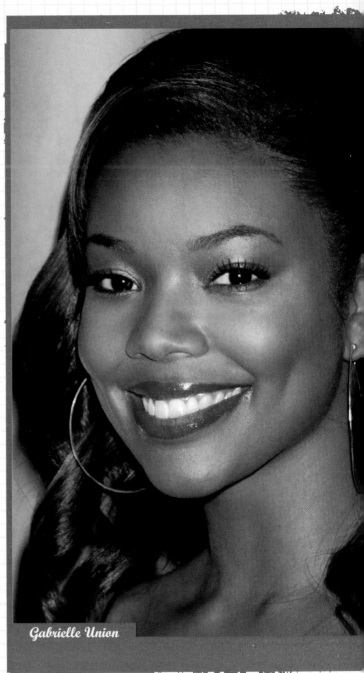

Gabrielle Union

3. Natural Matte Lips

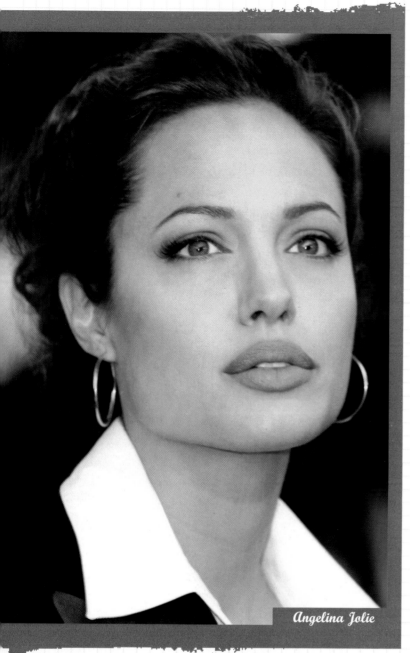

Angelina Jolie

THE LOOK: Natural matte lips, like Angelina Jolie's, are so hipster cool that people might even be a wee bit intimidated to talk to you, since you will be instantly transformed into a "cool girl."

WHAT IT'S GOOD FOR: Wear this look day or night when you want to feel like the hippest girl in the room. This works best when paired with natural-looking eye makeup.

What You'll Need
- [ ] LIP BALM
- [ ] FLESH-TONE LIP LINER
- [ ] LIP BRUSH
- [ ] MATTE FLESH-TONE LIPSTICK
- [ ] CLEAR GLOSS (OPTIONAL)

How To Get The Look

1. Since matte lips can be drying, before applying a matte lipstick, condition your kisser with an emollient balm so it's chap- and flake-free. If dead skin still lingers, gently exfoliate with a warm, wet wash cloth, which you can wipe back and forth over your lips for about 30 seconds. (Warning: if you do it for too long, you might irritate your lips.)

2. So the look is neat and stays put, line and fill in your lips with a light brown to nude lip pencil (let your skin tone be your guide—the key here is to have it match your skin tone as closely as possible). "Use your finger to blend color inward and blur lines," says Redleaf.

3. Using a lip brush (for more info on makeup brushes, see "Tools of the Trade" on page 54), apply a matte lip color that blends into your natural skin tone.

4. If the matte look is a little harsh to your taste, "try adding some gleam with a layer of clear gloss," says Redleaf.

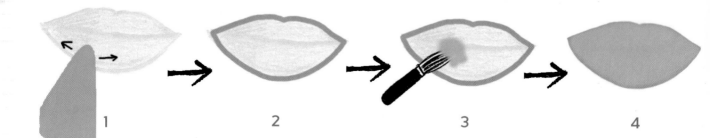

OUR ALL-TIME FAVORITE CELEB MAKEUP LOOKS

The next 10 pages are where you get to put everything you've learned about eyes, cheeks, glowing skin and color galore together! It was really hard to pick just 10, but here are our all-time favorite makeup looks. How'd we come up with them? We'll let you in on a little secret—we've been stalking your favorite celebs at all the cool parties, movie premieres, video shoots, and awards shows wearing makeup looks that are so out-of-this-world gorgeous that we had to get the scoop for you. From Mischa Barton's fantastic natural look to Beyoncé's golden sparkle, there's bound to be a look you'll want to try tonight. Celebrity makeup artists give you step-by-step instructions on how to make yourself up like a star.

Why We Love It
Beyoncé's golden glow is 24-carat glamorous.

What You'll Need
- [ ] LIQUID FOUNDATION
- [ ] EYE SHADOW BRUSH
- [ ] GOLD GLITTERY POWDER EYE SHADOW
- [ ] DARK BROWN EYELINER PENCIL
- [ ] COTTON SWABS
- [ ] BLACK CURLING MASCARA
- [ ] BLUSH BRUSH
- [ ] GOLD LUMINESCENT POWDER BLUSH
- [ ] CLEAR LIP GLOSS THAT'S INFUSED WITH GOLD

How To Get The Look
SKIN: Put a nickel-sized drop of foundation in the palm of your hand. With the pointer finger of your other hand, pick up a dab of foundation and tap the smallest possible amount onto problem areas, such as pimples and dark under-eye circles. Tap the foundation into the spots that need coverage until it disappears into your skin. Be careful not to rub the foundation into your skin with a back and forth motion—or you might just wipe it off. The idea here is to cover up the imperfection with the smallest amount of product.

EYES: "Use an eye shadow brush to apply gold glittery powder eye shadow to your upper lid, blended from lash line to just through the crease, so it fades as it rises," says Mally Roncal, one of Beyoncé's fave makeup artists. Line upper and lower lash lines with a dark brown eye pencil; use a cotton swab to blur the line on the upper lash line so it looks soft. Leave the lower line alone, so it stays neat. Deck top and bottom lashes with a black curling mascara, giving uppers two coats and lowers one coat.

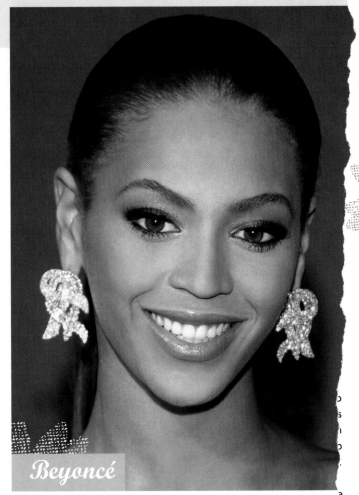

Beyoncé

CHEEKS: "Cast your cheeks in a golden glow with a gold-based powder blush," says Roncal; apply it to the apples of your cheeks with a blush brush.

LIPS: "Carry through that 24-carat sparkle with a gloss packed with gold shimmer," says Roncal.

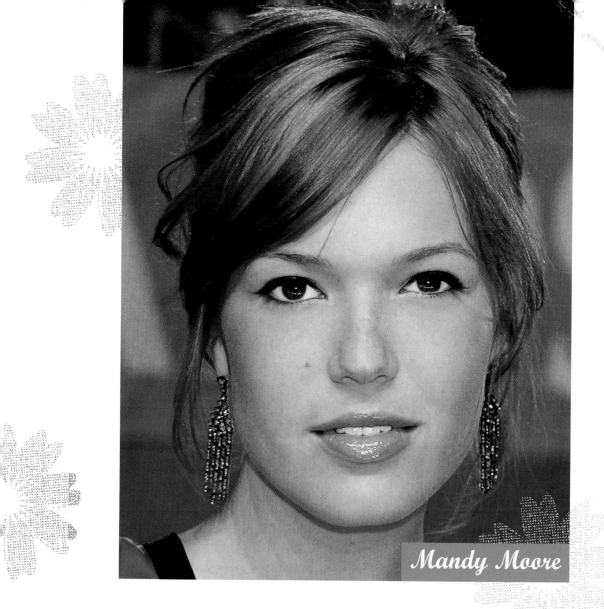

Mandy Moore

Why We Love It

Mandy's wearing similar peach colors on all of her features, but adds some sizzle with different textures, including frost and gloss.

What You'll Need

- [ ] LIQUID FOUNDATION
- [ ] EYE SHADOW BRUSH
- [ ] COTTON SWABS
- [ ] PALE PEACH FROSTY POWDER EYE SHADOW
- [ ] DARK BROWN MASCARA
- [ ] BLUSH BRUSH
- [ ] PEACH SHIMMERY POWDER BLUSH
- [ ] GLOSSY PEACH LIPSTICK

How To Get The Look

SKIN: Put a nickel-sized drop of foundation in the palm of your hand. With the pointer finger of your other hand, pick up a dab of foundation and tap the smallest possible amount onto problem areas, such as pimples and dark under-eye circles. Tap the foundation until it fades into your skin. If you rub the foundation into your skin, you will most likely wipe away the product and need to apply more. The idea here is to cover up imperfections with the smallest amount of product.

EYES: "Make your eyelids sparkle with a frosty pale peach powder eye shadow, applied with an eye shadow brush from lash line to just through the crease, so that it fades as it rises," says makeup artist Troy Surratt, who glams up celebs galore, including Mandy Moore, Hilary Duff, Mary-Kate and Ashley Olsen, and Amanda Bynes. Use a cotton swab to line your lower lash line, all the way from the inner corner to the outside corner, with the same shadow. Contining to use the same cotton swab, apply the shadow all the way around your inside corners, "so your tear duct area glows with peach," says Surratt. Softly emphasize your upper lashes with one coat of dark brown mascara. Leave lower lashes bare.

CHEEKS: Dress up your complexion with a pale peach powder blush that is packed with light reflective shimmer. Apply it with a blush brush to your cheek apples and blend up and out toward your temples.

LIPS: "Coat your lips with a super shiny peach lipstick," says Surratt.

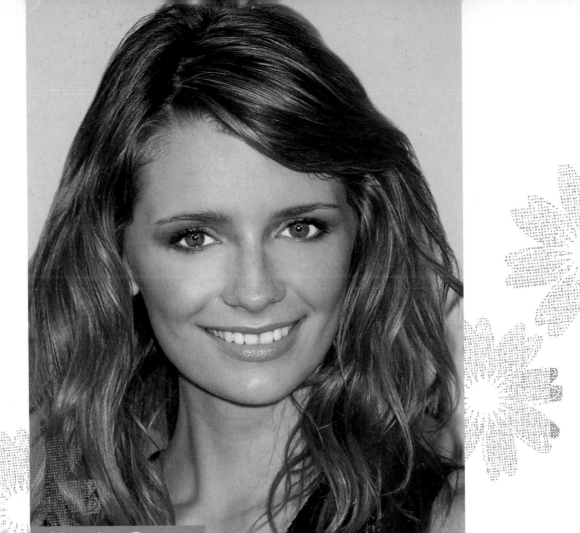

Mischa Barton

Why We Love It

Mischa's barely-there beauty, with softly sparkling eyes and cool natural lip color, steals the spotlight.

What You'll Need

- ❏ LIQUID FOUNDATION
- ❏ EYE SHADOW BRUSH
- ❏ COTTON SWABS
- ❏ EYELASH CURLER
- ❏ BEIGE POWDER EYE SHADOW
- ❏ LIGHT BROWN POWDER EYE SHADOW
- ❏ WHITE EYELINER PENCIL
- ❏ BLACK EYELASH TINT
- ❏ BLUSH BRUSH
- ❏ LIGHT BROWN-PINK POWDER BLUSH
- ❏ LIP PENCIL THAT MATCHES YOUR NATURAL LIP COLOR

How To Get The Look

SKIN: Put a nickel-sized drop of foundation in the palm of your hand. With the pointer finger of your other hand, pick up a dab of foundation and tap the smallest possible amount onto problem areas, such as pimples and dark under-eye circles. Tap the foundation until it fades into your skin. If you rub the foundation into your skin, you will most likely wipe away the product and need to apply more. The idea here is to cover up the imperfection with the smallest amount of product.

EYES: Bring out the shape of your eyes with a beige powder eye shadow. Apply it with an eye shadow brush to the lash line and blend up through the crease so it fades as it rises. Then, use a cotton swab to line your upper lash line with a light brown powder shadow. "To make the whites of your eyes look brighter, line the inside rim of your lower lash line with a white eyeliner pencil," says Surratt. Curl upper lashes and deck them with one coat of black eyelash tint, which adds color, not volume. Leave lower lashes bare.

CHEEKS: For a natural-looking flush, "use a blush brush to apply a light brown-pink powder blush to your cheek and blend up and out toward your temples," says Surratt.

LIPS: Use a lip pencil that matches your lip color to line and fill in your mouth. "Then blend it in with your finger toward the center of your mouth, so it looks like your natural lips, only better," says Surratt. This will add definition to your lip shape without looking like you have any lip color on.

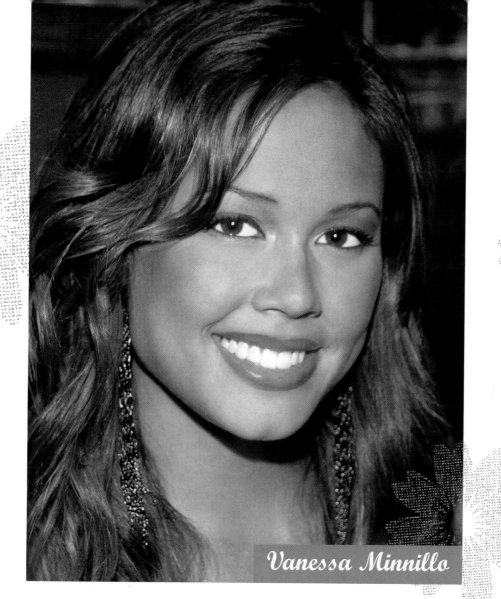

Vanessa Minnillo

Why We Love It

Vanessa's makeup looks subtly sexy since her natural shades—for eyes, cheeks and lips—are fancied up with shimmery finishes.

What You'll Need

- ❏ LIQUID FOUNDATION
- ❏ EYE SHADOW BRUSH
- ❏ COPPER POWDER EYE SHADOW
- ❏ BLACK EYELINER PENCIL
- ❏ BLACK MASCARA
- ❏ BLUSH BRUSH
- ❏ SHIMMERY BRONZE POWDER BLUSH
- ❏ LIP PENCIL THAT MATCHES YOUR NATURAL LIP COLOR
- ❏ CREAM LIPSTICK THAT'S ONE SHADE DARKER THAN YOUR NATURAL LIP COLOR
- ❏ SHIMMERY CLEAR LIP GLOSS

How To Get The Look

SKIN: Put a nickel-sized drop of foundation in the palm of your hand. With the pointer finger of your other hand, pick up a dab of foundation and tap the smallest possible amount onto problem areas, such as pimples and dark under-eye circles. Tap the foundation onto your little imperfections until it fades into your skin. If you rub the foundation into your skin, you will most likely wipe away the product and need to apply more. The idea here is to cover up imperfections with the smallest amount of product.

EYES: "Apply a copper powder eye shadow using an eye shadow brush to your upper lid, from lash line to crease," says Surratt. "With a black eyeliner pencil, thickly line your upper lash line—right above your lashes—and the inside rim of your lower lash line," says Surratt. Deck top and bottom lashes with two coats of black mascara. Give the outside section of your upper lash line two more coats.

CHEEKS: "To make your cheeks really stand out, apply a shimmery bronze powder blush to your cheek apples. Sweep it up and out toward your temple," explains Surratt.

LIPS: To complement—not compete against—your copper lids, line your lips with a lip pencil that matches your natural lip tone. Coat your lips with a cream lipstick that's one shade darker than your natural lip color. Top with "a clear lip gloss that's packed with silver shimmer," says Surratt.

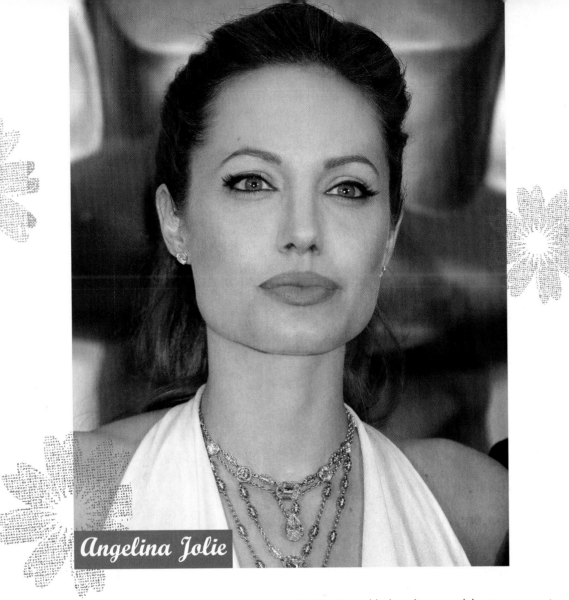

Angelina Jolie

Why We Love It

Angelina's black-rimmed eyes look so sexy and mysterious against her glowing skin.

What You'll Need

- ❏ TINTED MOISTURIZER
- ❏ BLACK EYELINER PENCIL
- ❏ EYELASH CURLER
- ❏ BLACK CURLING MASCARA
- ❏ PINK GEL BLUSH
- ❏ FLESH-TONE SHEER LIP GLOSS

How To Get The Look

SKIN: "Make your skin look wonderfully dewy with a tinted moisturizer," says Lamas. Apply it with your fingers in a thin layer all over your face.

EYES: "Use a black eyeliner pencil that is not too pointy—lightly tap the point on the back of your hand to dull the point—to line the inner rim of your upper and lower lash lines, all the way from the outside corner to the inside corner," explains Lamas. "To make your eyes look wide open, curl your upper lashes with an eyelash curler, then "apply black mascara to upper and lower lashes," he adds. Give your upper lashes two coats; give lower lashes just one to avoid unsightly smudging.

CHEEKS: Use a gel blush. It will go on nicely over the moisturizer. Take the smallest dab of gel with your middle finger and make three dots on your cheek, beginning just below your cheek apple and heading up and out toward your temple. Then, "blend up and out toward your temples," says Lamas.

LIPS: Since your skin and eyes are the main focus of this look, keep your lips simple with a sheer flesh-tone lip gloss.

Kate Hudson

Why We Love It

Kate's bold pink lips and shimmery lids are totally wearable—even off the red carpet.

What You'll Need

- ❏ TINTED MOISTURIZER
- ❏ BLACK LIQUID EYELINER
- ❏ OFF-WHITE CREAM EYE SHADOW
- ❏ BLACK CURLING MASCARA
- ❏ BABY PINK CREAM BLUSH
- ❏ BRIGHT PINK LIPSTICK
- ❏ BRIGHT PINK LIP LINER THAT MATCHES YOUR LIPSTICK

How To Get The Look

SKIN: Make your skin look even and splotch-free with a tinted moisturizer. Apply with your fingers in a thin layer all over your face.

EYES: Brighten up your eyelids with an off-white cream eye shadow, applied from lash line and blended up through the crease. Then, "apply a black liquid eyeliner in a very thin line above your upper lashes and extend it just beyond the outside corner of your eye," says Surratt. It's easier to make the line neat if you gently pull the corner of your eye near your temple taut with one hand, so your eyelid's surface is smooth. Apply liner with your free hand. Deck upper lashes with two coats of black curling mascara. Leave lower lashes bare.

CHEEKS: "Make your cheeks look like they are sweetly blushing by applying a baby pink cream blush to your cheek apples," says Surratt. Blend up toward your temples.

LIPS: Since this look is so focused on lips, apply color carefully so yours don't look messy. "First line and then fill them in with a bright pink lip liner that matches your lipstick exactly," says Surratt. Fill in with a glossy pink lipstick.

25 BEAUTY SECRETS EVERY STAR KNOWS

How do the stars stop their lipstick from smearing after a night of air-kissing on the red carpet? Do they ever get zits or do they know some cover-up secrets that the rest of us don't? Yes, if you study Hilary Duff, Liv Tyler, Cameron Diaz, or Jennifer Aniston, you'll learn that the reason they glow from within is that they have the best in the biz prepping their skin and applying their makeup. We grilled Hollywood's most sought-after makeup masters and collected their best tips and tricks. So even if you're just going to the mall, from now on, you'll always be ready for a close-up.

1. TRY BOLD COLOR. Madonna wears maroon mascara instead of black. It makes blue and green eyes really pop.

2. GET SHINY NAILS IN SECONDS. Beyoncé's nail technician at the The Paint Shop in Beverly Hills breaks a vitamin E capsule open and rubs the oil all over nails. This gentle vitamin oil moisturizes nails and cuticles so they'll look shiny—like you just applied a glossy topcoat.

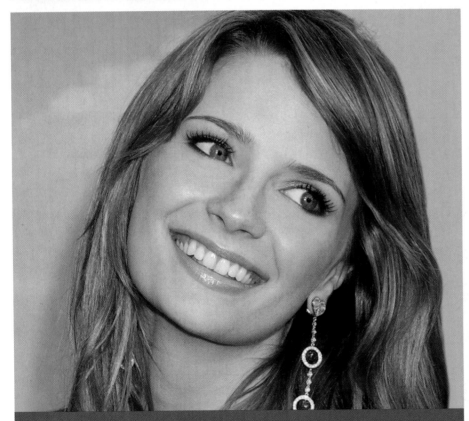

4. REDUCE CLUMPING MASCARA. Hollywood makeup artist Bryan Smoot uses this trick on **Mariah Carey**. If you feel like your mascara is looking too clumpy and unnatural, just grab a water spray bottle and lightly mist the wand of your mascara. Wait ten seconds and then apply the mascara to your lashes. The water dilutes the product just enough so that it leaves a little bit of color without the lumps. (This trick won't work with waterproof mascara.)

5. CLEAN YOUR NAILS WITH FACE TONER. If you're about to give yourself a manicure with polish, take this tip from **Uma Thurman's** nail guru. Before you apply any colored polish or base coat, swipe nails with a cotton ball that has been soaked in toner (the one you use on your face). This helps to remove any natural oils that are on the nails or residue from hand cream that keeps polish from sticking to your nails.

3. PERK UP A TIRED FACE. Hollywood makeup artist Agostina for Cloutier, who has worked with **Mischa Barton**, likes this simple and effective trick. First, apply powder blush on your cheeks, as usual. When you're done, rub the excess powder that's still on the brush over each eyebrow, starting from the brow bone and going up and out to the hairline. The color will be very subtle but it really brightens the skin and the eyes.

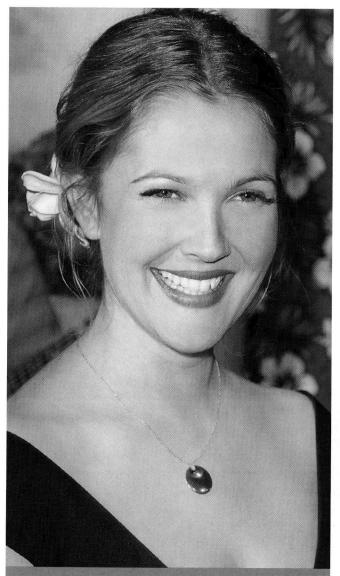

8. KNOW WHEN TO DITCH SPARKLY BRONZER. Makeup artist Sam Fine (he's worked with **Brandy**) cautions girls not to wear a bronzer with shimmery sparkles in it if they have pimples on their cheeks. Sparkles make acne stand out more. Instead, look for a powder formulation that is shimmer-free.

9. TONE DOWN RED LIPSTICK. If you just bought a new lipstick and feel like it's way too bright for you, try putting a touch of lipstick on the top of your hand and blending it with a tiny bit of foundation. This will soften the high-wattage shade a little bit. Use a lip brush to paint on your new hue.

10. SAY GOODBYE TO TAN LINES. If you're getting ready to go out after a day in the sun and notice that your bathing suit straps have created those oh-so-unattractive visible tan lines, don't worry. Fill them in with a bronzing powder. Instead of the big powder brush you use to apply it to your face, take a smaller eye shadow brush and use that to dust the powder along the lines.

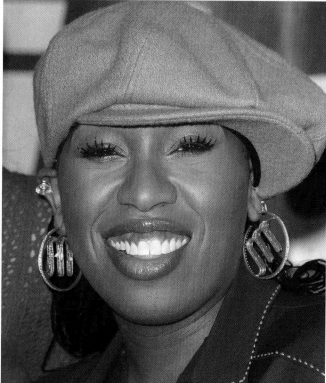

6. HOLD THAT LASH CURL. Hollywood makeup artist Bruce Grayson (who has worked with **Drew Barrymore**) says that curling your lashes is a great way to open up eyes without putting on any makeup. Try Grayson's trick of applying one coat of mascara and letting it set for a few seconds before curling. The first coat of mascara really helps the lashes to hold the curl. (To learn how to curl your lashes, check out "All Eyes on Hollywood," page 56.)

7. TAN LEGS IN A FLASH. Have you ever been on your way out the front door in shorts and looked down at your pale legs? No worries. If you don't have time to do a self-tanner, you can give skin a warm glow in a pinch by mixing loose bronzing powder with your body lotion. Mix the two up in the palm of your hand and blend up and down your legs, making sure not to let the lotion clump up in places like your ankles and knees.

11. LINE LIPS. Billy B., a makeup artist who regularly works with **Missy Elliott**, says to define your lips pick a pencil in a soft brown shade, line the lips, and then blend the color inward using a lip brush (this helps to soften the look). Afterward, apply your favorite lipstick or gloss.

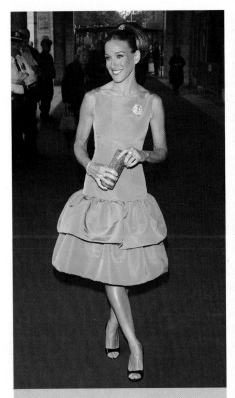

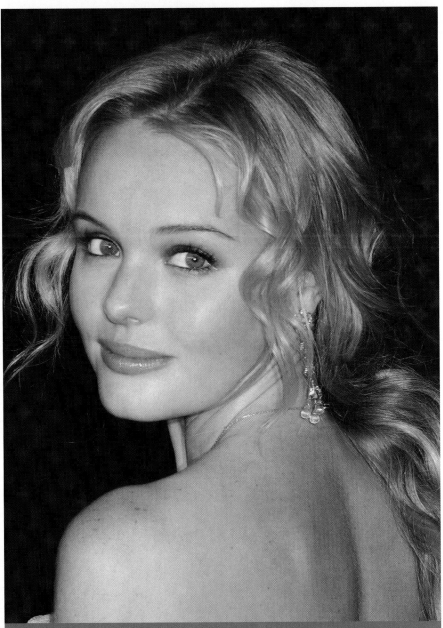

12. GRAB ATTENTION FOR YOUR LEGS. Sarah Jessica Parker does it by applying a shimmery body lotion on just the front part of her shins, from the ankles up to the knees. You can also dip a powder brush into a pot of loose shimmery powder and dust the same spots to get a similar effect.

13. LOOK GLAM "IN FIVE." Take a light-colored shimmery pencil (such as white for fair skin tones or gold for darker skin tones) and apply a small V right at the inner corner of the eye, with one side of the V going along the top eyelid while the other side goes along the bottom. The shimmery shade adds a dash of sparkle and, as an added bonus, also makes smaller eyes look larger.

14. SUBSTITUTE BLOTTERS. Hollywood makeup artist Sharon Gault, who works with stars like **Jennifer Garner** and **Kate Bosworth**, recommends blotting papers instead of powder for controlling a shiny T-zone, because they absorb shine without removing makeup. If you don't have any blotting papers on hand, just grab a facial tissue and peel apart the two sections of tissue so that you have two thin pieces. Use one of them to blot your face.

15. BUFF YOUR NAILS. What does **Tyra Banks** do when she doesn't have time for a total manicure? Gives her nails a quick buff. A nail buffer looks like a hard square sponge and can be found at the drugstore. Grab it in one hand and just brush it across the nails of the other hand in a quick back and forth motion. It keeps your nails natural but makes them look really shiny.

16. BRONZE THOSE BROWS. If you're African-American or Latina and love your brows, but wish they were a little lighter, here's a super-simple trick. Buy a bronze mascara and lightly brush over brows to tone them down. Everyone from **Beyoncé** to **Missy** has tried this.

17. GET A NATURAL LIP LOOK. At all the *Teen People* photo shoots, we notice that makeup artists often use their fingers to apply makeup instead of brushes. To get a lip look that looks really natural, take a lipstick and put a little bit of color on the tip of your index finger. Just tap the finger onto your lips and you're left with a pretty, subtle stain.

18. LET YOUR FINGERS DO THE BLENDING. Speaking of fingers, did you know that the reason it's so good to use them to apply cream products like blush and eyeliner is because the heat from your body makes it easier for the products to blend? But don't even think about touching your fingers to your face or your makeup without washing your hands with soap and warm water first.

19. STOCK UP ON SUPPLIES AT THE ART STORE. Hollywood makeup artists NEVER carry whole lipstick tubes. Instead, they'll hit an art-supply store and buy small, empty paint palettes. Once you have your palette, cut off the tips of your favorite lipsticks and put each shade in its own section of the palette. This way you can tote more than one shade at a time as well as mix up your own custom colors. Art stores are also great places to scope out paint boxes that can double as makeup boxes.

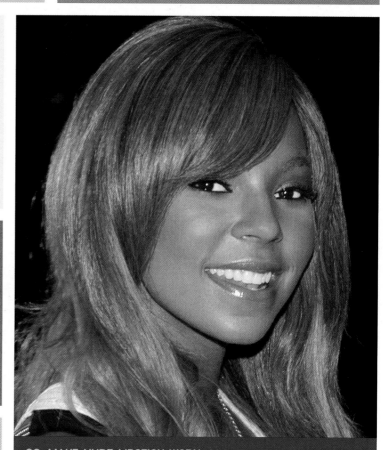

20. SAY GOODBYE TO RACCOON EYES. If you're using dark eye shadow, Billy B. suggests that you always apply the shadow before applying any concealer under the eyes. This is because small flecks of the shadow will most likely fall down and land just below your lower lashes while you're applying your eye shadow. After applying eye shadow, just take a moist cotton swab and wipe away any eye shadow that drifted downward. Then apply under-eye concealer for a clean look.

21. SWIPE A LIPSTICK ON YOUR LIDS. Makeup artist Steven Cooper, who has glammed up the likes of **Charlize Theron**, likes to use lip gloss as a quick get-glam trick for eyes. The best shade for every eye is a bronze shimmer gloss. Just apply a dab on your lid (right above your top lashes) and blend with your finger. The sparkles in the gloss will really accentuate your eyes. Add a coat of mascara and you're done.

23. MAKE NUDE LIPSTICK WORK. Makeup artist Ayako, who has worked on **Ashanti**, loves the look of beige or neutral-tone lips. If you are fair-skinned, look for a beige tone that has a bit of pink to it— otherwise you will look washed out. Those with darker skin tones shine with pure nude or brown shades but should pick one that has a hint of shimmer to it.

22. KNOW WHAT YOU REALLY LOOK LIKE IN YOUR MAKEUP. Do what the pros do and snap a picture of yourself. This is a great way to test if your foundation matches your skin tone or if that lipstick shade is too dark for you. This is great to do in the summer, when your skin may get a little bronzed from being outside. Your regular shades won't match your skin's new hue.

24. GET YOUR ROUTINE DOWN. All makeup artists we talked to say that you shouldn't be spending ages in front of the mirror every morning. Their suggested time? Seven minutes.

25. KNOW YOUR BEST BEAUTY ASSET. It's a great smile, of course! Don't forget to brush twice a day with a whitening toothpaste and you'll always be camera-ready.

FAST-FIX TRICKS

T hink celebs are totally satisfied with their looks? Think again. Just like you, stars like Reese Witherspoon, Gwen Stefani, and Monica may find themselves wishing they had a more even complexion, fuller lips, straighter teeth, or thicker brows. But just because you think you have a beauty concern doesn't mean the rest of the world sees it. As a matter of fact, it's just as likely your friends love the part of you that you wish you could change.

Bottom line, while it may be true that beauty is in the eye of the beholder–the most important "beholder" is the person who stares right back at you in mirror. And if you've got the urge to tweak what you see, the good news is: we've gathered a bunch of celebrity makeup pros who, with just a few swishes of a makeup brush, know exactly how to correct what you may see as little imperfections. Check out these fast fixes–straight from celebrity makeup artists to you–for five of the most common "fix-ations."

PROBLEM: YOUR SKIN TONE IS UNEVEN

SOLUTION: Use foundation that matches your skin tone exactly (for more info on foundation, flip to "Getting Gorgeous!" on page 44) to spot-treat imperfections. "There's no need to glob it all over your face," or you will draw more instead of less attention to your skin, says Genevieve.

What You'll Need
- ❏ FOUNDATION
- ❏ LOOSE TRANSLUCENT POWDER
- ❏ POWDER BRUSH
- ❏ OIL-FREE TINTED MOISTURIZER

How To Do It
1. Put a very small amount of foundation that matches your skin tone onto your middle finger and tap it onto problem zones—like around your nostrils, on your chin, or over zits—until it fades into your skin. You want to use the least amount possible to cover the area. When applying, tap, don't rub. If you do rub the foundation, you will most likely wipe it away in the process. (For more information on concealer, see "Getting Gorgeous! on page 47.)

2. "To make the foundation stay put all day, use a powder brush (for more info, see "Tools of the Trade" on page 54) to set it with a light dusting of loose translucent powder," says Genevieve, makeup artist to Liv Tyler and Kirsten Dunst. So you don't apply too much powder to your face, after dipping the brush into loose powder, give the handle a few taps to remove excess powder, then dust onto the area that is covered with foundation.

3. If your whole face seems like a blotch-fest, forget about steps one and two, and simply cover your entire face with a light film of tinted moisturizer. ""It'll look sheer and natural, but still offer some coverage," says Genevieve. Squirt a little bit of tinted moisturizer onto your pointer finger, then apply to your face section by section (your nose, right cheek, left cheek, forehead, and chin). Use downward strokes so the little hairs on your face lay down instead of stick out.

Anne Hathaway

PROBLEM: YOUR SKIN IS A TOUCH TOO PALE

SOLUTION: Go from ghostly to sun-kissed with a coppery flush, just like Anne Hathaway does.

What You'll Need
- ❏ LIQUID FOUNDATION
- ❏ COPPERY PINK POWDER BRONZER
- ❏ BLUSH BRUSH (SEE "TOOLS OF THE TRADE" ON PAGE 54 FOR MORE INFO)
- ❏ BOLD LIP COLOR, LIKE RED, IN A CREAMY FORMULA

How to Do It

1. Apply the smallest amount of liquid foundation necessary to cover up any uneven spots, like pimples and under-eye circles. The color of the foundation should not be darker than your natural skin tone (for more info on finding your perfect match, check out "Getting Gorgeous!" on page 44). Put a nickel-sized drop of foundation in the palm of your hand. With the pointer finger of your other hand, pick up a dab of foundation and tap the smallest possible amount onto problem areas, such as pimples and dark under-eye circles. Tap the foundation onto the problem area until it fades away into your skin. Do not rub the product, or you will just wipe it off and have to apply more. The idea here is to cover up the imperfection with the smallest amount of product.

2. Create a sun-kissed glow. "Use a blush brush to apply a coppery-pink powder bronzer to spots on your face that the sun hits when you are outside, like your forehead, nose, cheeks, chin, and eyelids," says Genevieve. "Carry the color down to your chest, shoulders, and collarbone" she adds, "if they will be showing, so you don't give away the fake-out."

3. Bold lips look hot against pumped-up pale skin. Try a bright red, rose, or berry lipstick. A gloss in these colors would also work. "Apply it to your lips very carefully," warns Genevieve; "since your skin is so fair, any messiness, like color outside the lines of your lips, will really stand out."

Gwyneth Paltrow

PROBLEM:
YOUR LIPS ARE ON THE SKINNY SIDE

SOLUTION: Plump up your pucker with a lip look that Angelina Jolie would envy!

What You'll Need:

☐ LIP-PLUMPING LIPSTICK OR LIP LINER IN A BOLD SHADE, LIKE BRIGHT PINK OR DEEP ROSE
☐ SHINY, OPAQUE LIP GLOSS OR LIPSTICK, IN THE SAME SHADE AS THE LINER (TIP: BUY THE SAME BRAND OF LIP LINER AND LIPSTICK SO COLORS WILL MATCH)
☐ CLEAR LIP GLOSS

How To Do It

1. In the past couple of years, tons of companies have come out with lipsticks packed with ingredients that are said to temporarily plump up your lips. All you have to do is carefully apply the lipstick to your lips, and they should plump up within a few minutes. But the results won't last forever, maybe just a few minutes. For longer-lasting results, try the following tips.

2. Make a half smile (no teeth showing—just make your lips taut so they're easier to line). Now "make your lips look bigger by carefully lining them just outside the rim with lip liner," says Jerrod Blandino, creator of Two Faced cosmetics and makeup artist to Gwen Stefani, Mary-Kate Olsen, Avril Lavigne, and Jessica Simpson. Start at the middle of your upper lip and draw your line out to the corner; then do the other side. Next, line the bottom lip, again just outside the rim, starting from the center and working out. Then use the liner to completely "color in" between the lines, covering your entire lip area.

3. Shine makes lips look fuller because light reflects off all the gloss. Use a lip brush (for more info on brushes, see "Tools of the Trade" on page 54) to precisely cover every bit of your lips plus the outside rim with lip gloss or shiny lipstick. Be extra careful about staying inside the lines.

4. To make lips look even larger, "fill in just the center of your lips with a clear gloss," says Blandino.

PROBLEM: YOUR LIPS ARE FULLER THAN YOU'D LIKE.

SOLUTION: Making your lips look less full is easy. It all comes to down to where you apply your lipstick. Blandino explains, "to make your lips look thinner, apply most of your lipstick or gloss in the middle part of your lips, like around where they come together instead of along the outer edges."

What You'll Need
- ❏ LIP PENCIL THAT MATCHES YOUR LIP COLOR
- ❏ LIPSTICK OR GLOSS IN THE COLOR OF YOUR CHOICE

How To Do It

1. Using a sharpened lip pencil that matches your natural lip color, "line just inside the outer rim of your upper and lower lips," says Blandino. For a neat, precise line, start on your upper lip in the center and make one line to the right corner, ending just inside the lip line. Go back to the center and do the same to the left corner.

2. Next, line the inside rim of your bottom lip from just inside the right corner all the way to the left corner. The idea here is to attract attention to the line you create inside your natural lip border, so lips look less full.

3. Use your finger to dab a lipstick or gloss of your choice (even if it comes in an easy-to-apply tube) and then tap the color onto the center of your lips and blend out to the edges. This way, "color will be heaviest and most noticeable in the middle—not the outskirts—of your mouth and the outer rim of your lips will look softer and fade away," says Blandino.

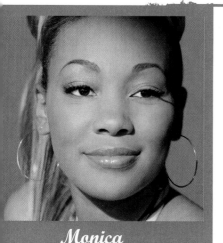

Monica

PROBLEM: YOUR EYEBROWS LOOK BARELY THERE

SOLUTION: Whether you over-plucked or were born with sparse brows, here's how to fake some fullness.

What You'll Need
- ❏ TWEEZERS WITH A SLANTED TIP (FOR PRECISE PLUCKING)
- ❏ EYEBROW BRUSH
- ❏ EYEBROW PENCIL

How To Do It

1. Random hairs may appear even on the skinniest brows. "You need to remove any strays below or between your brows with your tweezers, so they look neat," says Blandino. Tweezing hurts less if you tweeze in the direction your brow hairs grow.

2. Brush your brows up toward your forehead with an eyebrow brush—even a soft toothbrush will work. Neat brows are easier to work with.

3. Now pick up your eyebrow pencil—carrot tops and blonds, go for a shade that is one to two shades darker than your natural brow color; brunettes, choose a color one to two shades lighter than your natural color—and make sure it's been sharpened to a point.

4. Beginning near your nose, using short, feathery upward strokes, start filling in your brows. Make them thickest near your nose, then gradually thinner, switching to longer, downward feathery strokes as you reach the arch. Make them thinnest at the end. "That light, feathery touch is crucial so you don't overdo it and end up with fake-looking brows," says Blandino. Of course, the good news here is that if you don't like what you've done, you can wash it off and start all over. Practice makes perfect.

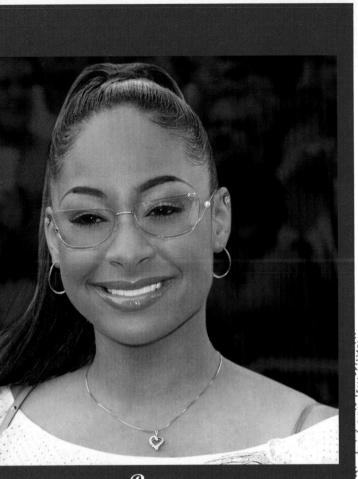

Raven

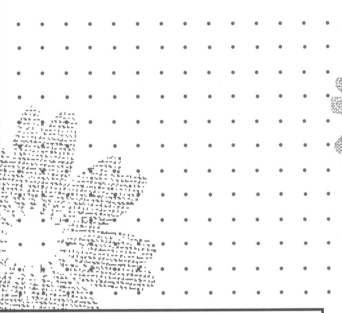

PROBLEM: YOU HATE YOUR GLASSES

SOLUTION: News flash: Glasses are a super-hip accessory—check out Raven's specs! Plus, the lenses actually enhance your beauty because they can magnify whatever makeup you have applied to your eyes. But you have to get your makeup right or you'll look a sight.

What You'll Need
- ❏ TWO SUBTLE POWDER EYE SHADOWS THAT ARE JUST A LITTLE BIT DARKER THAN YOUR SKIN TONE, ONE A SHADE DARKER THAN THE OTHER
- ❏ EYE SHADOW BRUSH
- ❏ EYELASH TINT (FOR MORE INFO ON LASH TINTS, CHECK OUT "GETTING GORGEOUS" ON PAGE 49)

How to Do It
1. Use an eye shadow brush to coat lids—from lash line to crease—with the powder eye shadow in the lighter shade. "Blend really well—if you don't, your glasses will magnify that you were sloppy," says Genevieve.

2. Use the eye shadow brush to line only the upper lash lines with the darker shade. "Don't use eyeliner pencils—they can look too bold magnified under your specs," warns Genevieve.

3. Use an eyelash tint to add color to upper lashes without upping volume. Too-long lashes will look clumpy and spidery under specs.

PROBLEM: YOU DON'T LIKE YOUR NOSE

SOLUTION: To draw attention away from your nose, play up another feature on your face, like your eyes, with a bright pop of your favorite color.

What You'll Need
- ❏ CONCEALER THAT MATCHES YOUR SKIN TONE
- ❏ POWDER EYE SHADOW IN A BRIGHT COLOR OF YOUR CHOICE, LIKE BLUE OR GREEN
- ❏ EYE SHADOW BRUSH
- ❏ VOLUMIZING MASCARA IN BLACK

How To Do It:

1. Since your eyes will be attention grabbers, disguise any dark under-eye circles with a concealer that matches your skin tone (for more info on concealers, check out "Getting Gorgeous!" on page 47). Use your middle finger to gently dab the color over any discoloration.

2. Dip the eye shadow brush into the powder shadow to pick up color, then sweep the brush over your lids, from lash line to crease. Color should be boldest near your lash line and fade as it rises up to the crease (for more info on eye shadow brushes, check out "Tools of the Trade" on page 54).

3. Deck top lashes with two coats of volumizing mascara.

PROBLEM: YOU'RE WEARING BRACES

SOLUTION: If you don't want your braces to stand out too much, coat your lips with natural-looking color and "keep them moist and healthy," says Genevieve—the more flaky they look, the more they will attract unwanted attention.

What You'll Need
- ❏ MOISTURIZING LIP BALM
- ❏ GLOSS OR LIPSTICK WITH BUILT-IN MOISTURIZERS
- ❏ 100 PERCENT PURE PETROLEUM JELLY
- ❏ SOFT, CLEAN WASHCLOTH

How to Do It

1. Apply a moisturizing lip balm containing SPF 15 to your kisser three times a day—morning, midday, and evening.

2. When picking lip colors, "go for glosses and lipsticks with built-in moisturizers and avoid matte lipsticks, which can be drying," says Genevieve. So your lips don't scream, "look at me, look at me!", pick shades that are similar to your natural lip color—an exact match or one shade lighter or darker (for more information on lip colors and formulations, see "Getting Gorgeous!" on page 52).

3. If your lips are flaky, exfoliate dead skin by coating lips with tons of 100 percent pure petroleum jelly, then gently rubbing back and forth with a clean, soft washcloth.

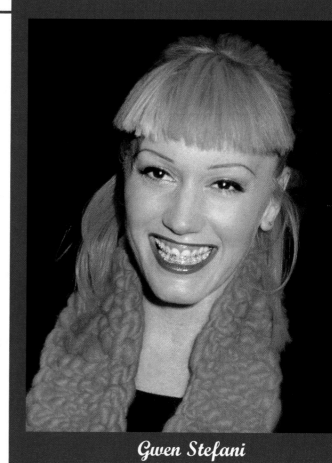

Gwen Stefani

ALL-NIGHT BEAUTY SECRETS

*J*t can really be a challenge to keep your makeup looking great when you're partying from dusk 'til dawn, like at prom. Even celebs don't seem to have the answer to party-proof makeup all the time and are occasionally caught looking less than perfect. As the hours go by, that look you so carefully created often fades—or smears and smudges. Especially when you're dancing—or kissing—the night away.

We've all been there. Your blush and lipstick vanish into thin air, while your eye makeup drips down your face. Not a pretty look—especially when some photographer is clicking away with a camera. To make sure that never happens to you, celebrity makeup artist Jim Crawford, who recently prettied up Anna Paquin for an all-night bash, gives you step-by-step instructions on how to apply makeup so it stays put all night long—no matter what your plans.

★ SECRET WEAPONS

Before you get started, here are three secret makeup weapons to keep your face in place. Celebs use this stuff all the time to make their makeup last and last. How do you think Gwen Stefani keeps lipstick on throughout her concerts?

MAKEUP PRIMER: This white or clear lotion is applied over moisturizer in a super thin film to even out the feel of your skin (so bumps are smoothed away as much as possible) and to make your makeup stay put longer. You put it on exactly like a moisturizer in a thin layer.

EYE MAKEUP PRIMER: This is just like a "makeup primer," but made in a more delicate formula for the sensitive skin around your eye. To apply, dab your index finger into the primer if it comes in a pot, or squirt a drop of primer onto your index finger if it comes in a tube, and tap primer over your eyelid, from lash line to eyebrow, until it blends into the skin.

LIP COLOR SEALANT: This clear liquid is put on over your lipstick in a thin film to lock on your color. You can apply it straight from the tube or with your finger.

LONG-LASTING PERFECT-LOOKING SKIN

Step 1: No makeup will stick to a face that is covered with dirt and oil, so wash your face with a gentle cleanser and lukewarm water; pat dry with a towel.

Step 2: To ready your skin for makeup, first apply an oil-free moisturizer, all over your face. Let it absorb into your skin for about 10 minutes; the primer won't work if your skin is oily.

Step 3: Apply the makeup primer (one of those three "secret weapons" we talk about in the box at left), which will smooth out your skin so makeup can go on easily.

Step 4: "The best way to make foundation last all night is to use the least amount you can, to achieve the desired effect, which is perfectly even-looking skin," says Crawford. Plus, pick formulations that say they are "long lasting" on the bottle. Don't use your finger to apply the foundation; it has oil on it that will mix with the product and make it fade faster. Instead, pour a nickel-sized drop of foundation onto your palm and dab it with the corner of a small wedge-shaped makeup sponge (for more info on sponges, see "Tools of the Trade" on page 54) picking up a very small amount of foundation with the tip of the sponge. Then tap the sponge only on the areas where you need a little coverage, such as redness around your nose, dark circles under your eyes, and to conceal pimples. Keep in mind, the more foundation you apply, the more likely it will come off, since thick layers are more likely to slip off your skin and smudge stuff, like your date's collar.

Step 5: "To keep your foundation from smudging or fading, give it a dusting of loose translucent powder," says Crawford. Dab a loose powder brush (for more info on brushes, see "Tools of the Trade" on page 54) into the powder pot, tap the handle of the brush against your palm to shake off excess powder—again, less is more—and dust powder on the spots where you applied foundation. This is called "setting your foundation," says Crawford.

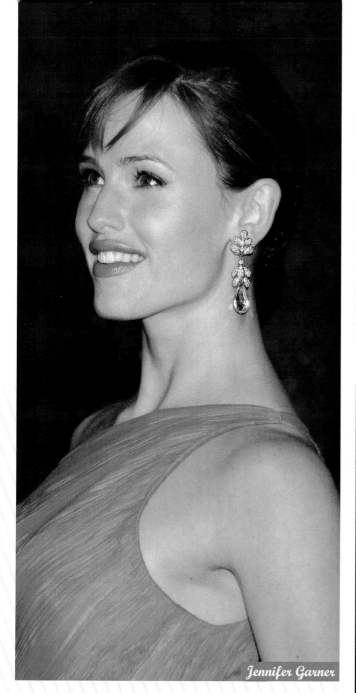

Jennifer Garner

LONG-LASTING LIPS

Step 1: Make sure your lips have a smooth surface and are free of any dry skin and flakes by rubbing a warm, damp washcloth back and forth over them.

Step 2: Use a lip liner pencil to line and fill in your lips. Blot with a tissue. Line and fill them in a second time.

Step 3: "Next apply a long-lasting cream lipstick," recommends Crawford. Don't glob it on; that approach won't make it last longer. Instead, apply a thin layer, blot with a tissue, just like you did with the lip liner, and then apply another thin coat. Or opt for a lip tint, which stains your lips for long-lasting coverage.

Step 4: Top your lip color with a lipstick sealant, which is a clear film that helps your color stay put for hours—even if you get a good-night smooch!

Step 5: Top off the look with a thin layer of gloss. Think of it as one more bit of protective coating.

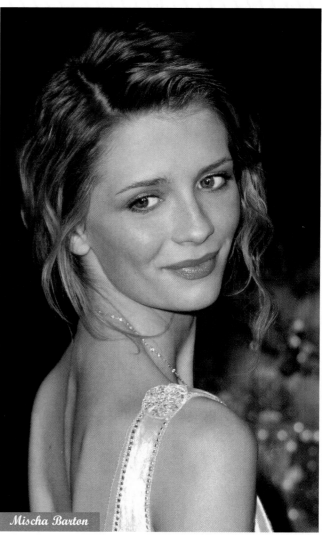

Mischa Barton

Step 6: To make your blush last all night, Crawford suggests, "pick a blush that is super see-through, like a gel, and one that has a strong color." (For more blush info, see "Getting Gorgeous!" on page 50.) This way, you will use less color to achieve the desired effect, but the color will be stronger; and, because it is put on in a thin film, it will last longer. A little colored gel can go a long way. "This time, you can use your fingers to apply; dab the gel onto your cheek apples and blend up and out toward your temple," says Crawford. Set with a light dusting of transparent loose powder, just like you did with your foundation spots. Dip the loose powder brush into the powder, then tap the handle to shake off excess powder and brush onto your cheeks and up toward your temples.

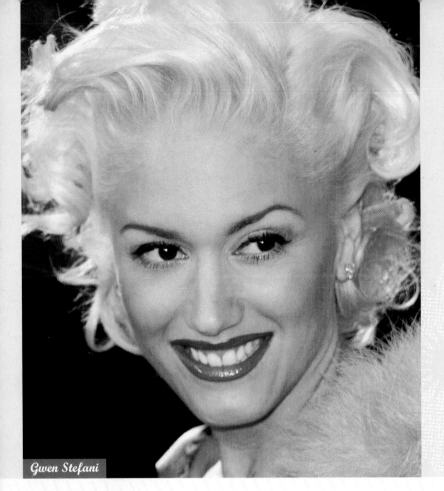

Gwen Stefani

AROUND-THE-CLOCK EYE MAKEUP

Step 1: To keep your eye makeup from running, coat your lids with either a transparent loose powder or eye make-up primer (see "Secret Weapons," page 84). "Both the primer and the powder will absorb any oils that are on your eyelids, which would otherwise cause makeup to slip," says Crawford. They will also create a smooth surface for easy makeup application.

Step 2: To prevent the dreaded raccoon eyes, "the key is to apply eye makeup only to your upper eyelid area," says Crawford. This may not seem like a good idea to you if you are used to wearing eye makeup on the lower lash line, but give it a try because it will look great and last all night.

Step 3: Use an eye shadow brush (for more info on brushes, see "Tools of the Trade" on page 54) to apply a powder shadow color of your choice over your eyelid, from your lash line up to the crease. Avoid using cream or gel eye shadows since they tend to melt and fade much fast than powder eye shadows. If you want your eye makeup to last, don't use your fingers, as the oils they hold will cover your lid and cause makeup to run.

Step 4: Then, use the same eye shadow brush to apply a powder eye shadow that is one shade darker than the eye shadow you just applied to your lid, to your crease. Place the bristles in your crease, which falls at the top of your eyeball, and sweep the brush back and forth, resting it on the ball. By accenting your crease, Crawford promises, "you will add enough definition to your eye area to compensate for leaving the lower lash line bare of any makeup."

Step 5: Set your eye makeup with translucent loose powder. Dip a loose powder brush into the powder, tap the handle against your palm to shake off any excess loose powder, and dust what remains on the brush over your closed eyelids.

Step 6: Deck top lashes only with two coats of waterproof mascara. Then add two more coats of the same mascara to the outside quarter of upper lashes, for a little more definition. Because those lashes will be a little longer than the rest, due to the extra coats of mascara, your eye will look super sexy.

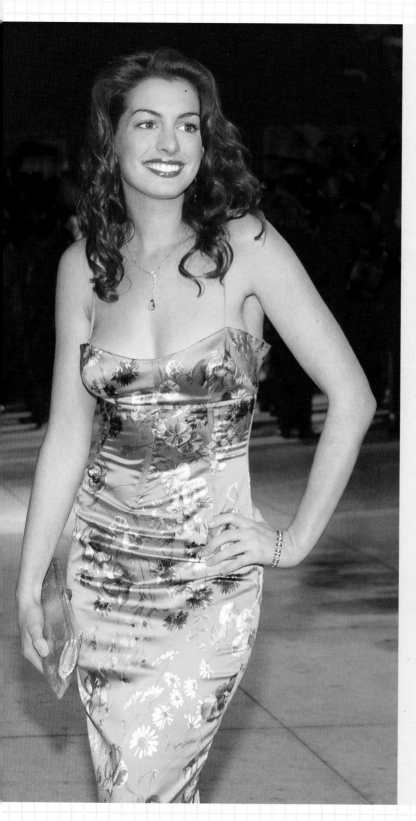

PROM PURSE ESSENTIALS

Arm yourself with these mini touch-up products and you'll be ready for any beauty emergency.

OIL-ABSORBING SHEETS—After dancing, sweat and oil can coat your face and melt makeup. To wipe away perspiration but keep your makeup intact, simply tap—don't rub—an oil-absorbing sheet over your face.

LIPSTICK OR GLOSS—The quickest and easiest way to brighten up a fading look is to swipe some color and shine over your lips.

DEODORANT WIPES—If you know you will be dancing a lot, stash some of these portable sheets in your bag to avoid underarm odor.

BREATH MINTS—Freshen up with breath mints before hitting the dance floor.

chapter four

HOLLYWOOD HAIR

the best tress secrets of the stars

QUIZ: HOW HAIR HIGH-MAINTENANCE ARE YOU?

Do you spend hours in the bathroom creating a masterpiece hairstyle every morning or are you the type of girl for whom two minutes is too long? Just like some stars always seem to be out and about with a perfectly undone 'do (think Mary-Kate and Ashley Olsen), others are always perfectly primped (Jennifer Lopez always looks camera-ready). The rest of us are exactly the same. Take this quiz and see if you're doing way too much or not enough when it comes to mastering your mane.

1. COULD YOU EVER LEAVE THE HOUSE WITHOUT BLOW-DRYING YOUR HAIR?

A) Never

B) Sure

C) On weekends

2. WHAT IS YOUR FAVORITE HAIR PRODUCT?

A) My shampoo/conditioner-in-one

B) My straightening iron

C) My expensive conditioner

3. HOW OFTEN DO YOU GO TO THE HAIR SALON?

A) Every 4–6 months

B) Every 2–3 months to touch up my roots

C) Once a year for a trim

4. WHAT WAS THE LAST THING YOU DID TO YOUR HAIR?

A) Tried an at-home hair color

B) Learned how to do a simple updo

C) Blew it straight and used a straightening iron

5. HOW MANY STYLING PRODUCTS DO YOU USE IN THE MORNING?

A) A mousse, hairspray, and pomade to make the ends piece-y

B) A gel and maybe some hairspray

C) I wash 'n' go

6. WHICH STAR'S STRAND STYLE DO YOU MOST ADMIRE?

A) Jennifer Lopez

B) Amanda Bynes

C) Kirsten Dunst

7. WHAT'S THE THING THAT BUGS YOU MOST ABOUT YOUR HAIR?

A) That it never quite looks how I want it to

B) That it sometimes gets frizzy

C) That I don't know what to do with it

8. HOW LONG HAVE YOU HAD YOUR CURRENT HAIRSTYLE?

A) I've always had longish hair

B) I keep the cut but love to color it and change styles

C) I just chopped some cool longish bangs

9. WHAT'S YOUR FAVORITE GLAM UPDO?

A) Something Jessica Simpson-esque with lots of curls

B) A classic twist in the back, perhaps with a cool accessory

C) The front pulled back and the rest hanging down

10. WHICH ONE OF BEYONCÉ'S HAIRSTYLES DO YOU LIKE THE BEST?

A) When it's long and curly

B) When it's pulled back in a classic pony

C) The amazing updos

YOUR SCORE

1. A=1 B=3 C=2 | 2. A=3 B=1 C=2 | 3. A=2 B=1 C=3 | 4. A=2 B=3 C=1 | 5. A=1 B=2 C=3

6. A=1 B=3 C=2 | 7. A=1 B=3 C=2 | 8. A=3 B=1 C=2 | 9. A=1 B=2 C=3 | 10. A=2 B=3 C=1

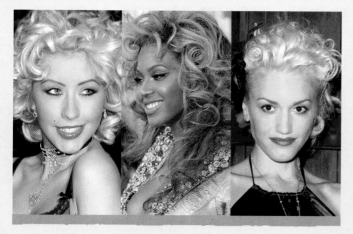

10–16, High-Maintenance Mane

STARS WHOSE STRANDS YOU LOVE:
Christina Aguilera, Beyoncé, and Gwen Stefani

You are a total expert when it comes to your locks—just make sure you're not doing too much. Does it take you more than two styling products to get out the door in the morning? Hollywood stylists say any more than that and you might be trying to coax your tresses into a style that goes against your hair type. If you have curly hair and spend an hour blowing it straight every morning, try something different—learn to work with the curls or ask a stylist about chemical straightening. And make sure to pamper your hair so it stays in good shape. Use a mild shampoo daily and switch to a clarifying shampoo once a week to thoroughly wash out residue from your styling stuff (these shampoos are a bit drying so you don't want to use them too often).

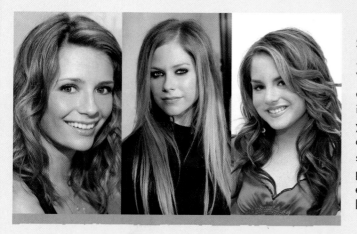

17–24, Manageable Mane

STARS WHOSE STRANDS YOU LOVE:
Mischa Barton, Avril Lavigne, and JoJo

You spend some mirror time getting your locks just so, but it's not a lengthy process. Some days you feel like making the effort and busting out the blow-dryer, but other days, you'll rock a ponytail. Next time you have a hair appointment, ask your stylist what products he recommends just to be sure you're on the right track. Ever tried a shine spray, styling wax, or straightening balm? Switching to the right product can shave even more minutes off your styling routine. Also, experiment with some cute hair accessories. Even a basic ponytail can look unique with a cool clip.

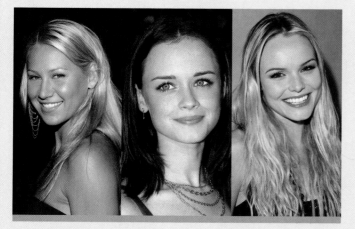

25–30, Minimalist Mane

STARS WHOSE STRANDS YOU LOVE:
Anna Kournikova, Alexis Bledel, and Kate Bosworth

There's nothing wrong with being relaxed about your strands, but it's also fun to experiment with different styles every once in a while. Check out "Our Top 10 Hairstyles" on page 102 or just grab the latest *Teen People* to see what the stars are doing. There are really easy ways to update your look—it can be as easy as moving your ponytail from the nape of your neck to the top of your head. When it comes to products, make sure you're using the right ones for your hair type, especially shampoo and conditioner—volumizing shampoo and conditioner are great for fine, straight hair but will wreak havoc on very curly hair. Next time you get a trim, ask the stylist how to do a basic blow-dry. That way you'll know how to get it looking good when you need to.

THE ULTIMATE HAIR TYPE GUIDE

There's nothing quite as glam as gorgeous hair. Celeb strands always seem to be so shiny, so perfectly straight or curled and healthy. How do they do it? We'll let you in on a little secret: stars have bad hair days too. But celebs also have a secret weapon–hair stylists on call 24/7. Here, celebrity hair stylists tell you what to do–and not to do–to make sure your hair always looks its best.

FINE & STRAIGHT HAIR

YOU HAVE FINE, STRAIGHT HAIR IF . . .

*Your hair falls flat unless you really make an effort to give it some volume, such as blowing it dry with your head upside down the whole time—and then it droops by third period anyway.

*A shampoo only keeps the greasies at bay for a day; by the next morning, your scalp and roots look and feel oily.

*Conditioner and styling products usually weigh your hair down and can even make it look dirty, so you often bag them entirely.

FINE & STRAIGHT HAIR DOS

- GIVE YOUR HAIR BODY AND SHINE WITH THE RIGHT CUT. If you have a heart, square, or round face shape, "try a cut with a strong shape, like a bob with a few face-framing pieces for added lift," says celeb stylist Sally Hershberger, who works on famous locks galore, including Mandy Moore, Sarah Jessica Parker, and Renee Zellweger. Long bangs look great if you have a long face. An ideal length for you is between your chin and shoulders, since your tresses appear thinner as they grow longer.

- KEEP YOUR HAIR LOOKING GOOD–AND KEEP THIN, SCRAG-GLY-LOOKING ENDS AT BAY–with a strong, neat shape by getting trims every six weeks. This way, your hair will stay looking as thick at the ends as possible.

- WASH YOUR HAIR WITH A VOLUMIZING SHAMPOO EVERY DAY (hairdresser-speak for shampoos that help make your hair look thicker). "Use your fingers to work the shampoo into your scalp, to get your roots squeaky clean and the blood flowing," says Hershberger.

- CONDITION YOUR HAIR, IF YOU NEED TO, WITH A PRODUCT ESPECIALLY FOR FINE HAIR–it'll say so on the package. "To avoid weighing your hair down with product, just apply conditioner to the ends and avoid the roots at all costs," says celebrity stylist Brian Magallones, who works on Mischa Barton and Kelly Clarkson.

- USE VOLUMIZING PRODUCTS WHEN STYLING TO BOOST BODY. "Lightweight mousses (which look and feel like whipped cream) and volumizing sprays (which make hair seem thicker) are good options and can be applied directly to your roots, like you are spraying it onto your scalp, to add big-time lift to tresses," says Magallones.

- BLOW-DRY WITH YOUR HAIR UPSIDE DOWN, "using your fingers to lift your hair up and away from your scalp," says Magallones. Then flip upright for the last bit, using a big round brush to neaten the style and add extra volume.

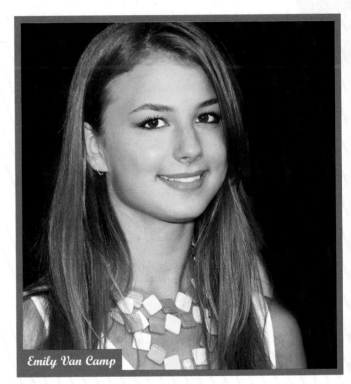

Emily Van Camp

FINE & STRAIGHT HAIR DON'TS

- LET A STYLIST USE A RAZOR TO CUT YOUR HAIR into "super-wispy styles with tons of layers, or your hair will have major frizz and flyaway issues, plus it will make your hair look even thinner," says Magallones.

- "LET YOUR HAIR GROW TOO LONG or it will get really stringy, thanks to weaker broken ends," says Ian James, hairstylist to such stars as Scarlett Johansson and Jennifer Love Hewitt. Also, your tresses will fall flat and drag down your face.

- WASH YOUR TRESSES WITH SHAMPOOS MADE FOR NOR-MAL, THICK, OR DRY HAIR. They are too heavy and will weigh your hair down.

- STYLE YOUR HAIR WITH HEAVY PRODUCTS, like creams, lotions, jellies, waxes, or pomades, "which will make your hair look dirty and flat," warns Magallones. Even too much silicone will weigh you down, so beware of products with that, too!

- TURN YOUR HAIR-DRYER ONTO HIGH. That degree of intense heat can burn and dry out your delicate tresses. "Stick to the medium heat setting," recommends Hershberger.

THICK & STRAIGHT HAIR

YOU HAVE THICK, STRAIGHT HAIR IF . . .

*You can get a big elastic band around your ponytail no more than twice.

*After shampooing, you hair keeps looking and feeling clean for up to three days unless you've worked up a sweat working out or playing sports.

*All you do is comb your hair after a shower and it dries stick-straight—even if you don't apply any hair product.

THICK & STRAIGHT HAIR DOS

- GIVE YOUR HEAVY HAIR BODY AND BOUNCE by having your hairdresser use a razor (instead of scissors) to cut it into soft layers, which fall either above the chin or below the shoulder in length," recommends Hershberger. If you have an oval face, bangs can also lighten up your tresses. Layers that bounce outward look pretty on a heart-shaped face. Square and round faces look best with hair curled inward.

- SHAMPOO YOUR HAIR AS NEEDED, every two to three days, with a shampoo that is made for your hair type, whether that is dry or normal. "Really focus on the roots and scalp, which can be forgotten under all that hair," says Magallones.

- CONDITION YOUR HAIR EVERY TIME YOU SHAMPOO, "applying extra conditioner to the ends," recommends Magallones.

- "USE STYLING PRODUCTS THAT ARE LIGHTWEIGHT AND BODY-BUILDING, like gels and lotions, which you can apply to roots, then work down your hair with a wide-tooth comb," says Hershberger. Tip: If it is hard to work product through your thick hair, dilute it with a bit of water.

- "FLIP YOUR HEAD OVER AND BLOW-DRY YOUR HAIR ON HIGH HEAT, using your fingers to move roots up and away from your scalp until hair is halfway dry, then flip upright and use a paddle brush and pull two-inch sections out and under for a neat style," explains Magallones. Or, air-dry for a more natural look.

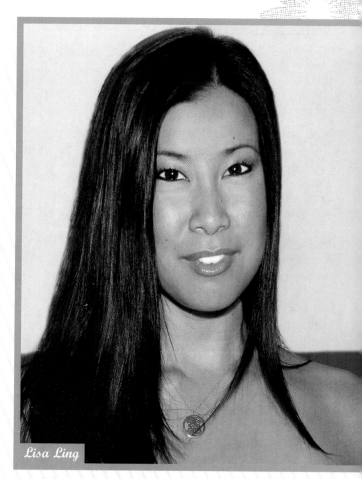

Lisa Ling

THICK & STRAIGHT HAIR DON'TS

- CUT YOUR HAIR INTO A BLUNT CHIN-LENGTH BOB WITHOUT LAYERS. Layers can look too severe and pouf out.

- LET YOUR HAIR GROW INDEFINITELY. "You will lose the shape, and your hair will look totally heavy and overwhelm your face," says Hershberger.

- GLOB CONDITIONER ONTO YOUR ROOTS. Using too much conditioner will weigh your hair down, so stick to applying it from halfway down the hair shaft to the ends.

- USE HEAVY STYLING PRODUCTS, like pomades and creams. They will just make your hair heavier.

- BLOW-DRY HAIR WITH IT UPRIGHT THE WHOLE TIME—IT WILL FALL FLAT. Also avoid using a round brush, which can bring on a tangled disaster.

FINE-WAVY OR FINE-CURLY

YOU HAVE FINE-WAVY OR -CURLY HAIR IF . . .

*When you let your hair dry naturally after only a single comb-through, it coils up into either tight or loose tendrils.

*Your hair needs to be washed every other day or it looks and feels greasy on and just around your scalp.

*When you brush your tresses after they are dry, you have a frizzfest on your hands.

FINE-WAVY OR -CURLY HAIR DOS

- "BRING OUT THE SHAPE OF WAVES AND CURLS, plus add volume, with the right cut, which is lots of layers—all over your head—with blunt ends," says Magallones. If you have a round or square face, go for layers around the face that curl toward your face. For a heart-shaped face, chin-length layers that curl outward look best. Long coiling bangs look perfect draping down a square-shaped face. When cutting layers, make sure your stylist uses scissors (not a razor) to cut blunt ends.

- "GET YOUR TRESSES CUT WHEN YOUR HAIR IS DRY so your stylist can see the natural ebb and flow of your curls and waves and work with them," says James.

- "SHAMPOO THIN TENDRILS ONLY AS NEEDED (when the grease starts showing, maybe every other day)," says Magallones.

- CONDITION HAIR EVERY TIME YOU WASH with a conditioning product made for fine hair, so it doesn't weigh down your locks.

- MAKE CURLS AND WAVES SPRING INTO SHAPE WITH A CURL-ENHANCING MOUSSE (a mousse looks and feels like whipped cream), "which you can apply from roots to tips of towel-dried hair," says Hershberger.

- COMB A STYLING PRODUCT THROUGH YOUR HAIR with a wide-toothed comb. Let hair air-dry so your spirals form naturally.

- POLISH YOUR MANE WITH A SHINE-ENHANCING SPRAY SERUM, which you first spritz in your palms, then rub onto the ends of tresses after hair is dry.

FINE-WAVY OR -CURLY HAIR DON'TS

- LEAVE YOUR HAIR ALL ONE LENGTH. "You can end up your looking like you have a pyramid-shaped head," warns Hershberger. If you have an oval- or square-shaped face, opt for shorter layers; for a round face, long layers look pretty.

- GO WITHOUT A TRIM FOR MORE THAN SIX WEEKS. Your curls and waves will be weighed down and will lose their oomph. Also, your hair can start to look a bit messy.

- APPLY CONDITIONER DIRECTLY TO YOUR ROOTS. They will collapse and can look greasy; instead, Magallones says, "apply conditioner halfway down your hair shaft to the ends."

- TRY TO BLOW-DRY HAIR. You will create a frizzy mess. If you simply must get your tresses dry ASAP, use a diffuser (an attachment that looks like a loudspeaker, and should have come with your dryer).

- "SPRAY PRODUCT DIRECTLY ONTO YOUR HAIR," says James. Instead, spray product into your hands, then rub it over your hair—fine hair will be weighed down by too much product sprayed on directly. Also, if too much product gets on curls, they'll be lost.

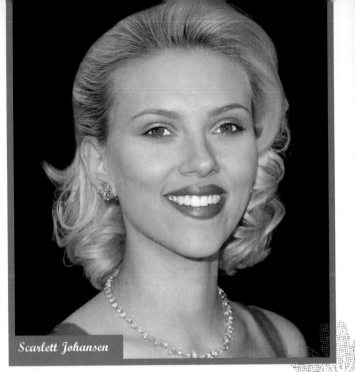

Scarlett Johansen

THICK-WAVY OR THICK-CURLY HAIR

YOU HAVE THICK-WAVY OR -CURLY HAIR IF . . .

*When you let your hair air-dry, curls and waves form naturally.

*You can go days on end—at least three—without shampooing tresses before your scalp starts to look and feel oily.

*Keeping your strands from becoming dry and strawlike is a constant battle, especially at the ends, which tend to fray a bit if you wait too long for a trim.

THICK-WAVY OR -CURLY HAIR DOS

- "CUT YOUR HAIR INTO LONG, CASCADING LAYERS ALL OVER YOUR HEAD, including sides, top, and back, to bring out your natural texture and lighten up the weight of all of your hair," says Hershberger. If you have an oval or square face, opt for shorter layers; for a round-shaped face, long layers look pretty.

- GET YOUR HAIR CUT AFTER IT'S AIR-DRIED. That way a stylist can see where your hair needs to be refined and each tendril can be cut individually, so your natural shape comes through.

- "WASH YOUR TRESSES WITH MOISTURIZING SHAMPOOS, since your hair tends to be dry," says James.

- CONDITION YOUR HAIR EVERY TIME YOU WASH WITH SHAMPOO or rinse with water, applying product from just below the roots to tips.

- "TREAT TRESSES TO A MOISTURIZING HAIR MASK ONCE A WEEK," says Hershberger. To give your tresses an all-out moisture surge, cover the mask with a shower cap and top with a towel that you have warmed in the dryer. The heat will turn the mask's moisturizing power up a notch or two.

- HAVE FUN WITH STYLING PRODUCTS TO GET THE MOST FROM YOUR MANE. To pump up your texture and style, try mixing equal parts styling gel and leave-in conditioner in the palm of your hand (about a quarter-sized dollop total), then apply from roots to tips of towel-dried hair.

- TAKE A BREAK FROM BLOW-DRYING EVERY SO OFTEN. "Let hair air-dry; while it's in the process, twist sections of hair around your finger (the smaller the section the tighter the curl and vice versa) to define waves and curls," says James.

- MAKE CURLS SHINE. Since curls can sometimes look dull, with a shine-enhancing serum. Rub a tiny bit between palms (you can always add more later) applied just below the roots all the way down to tips.

THICK-WAVY OR -CURLY HAIR DON'TS

- BAG THE LAYER IDEA COMPLETELY. As curls grow longer, they grow outward and you can end up looking like a triangle head. Plus, your face can look dragged down if your tresses are too heavy.

- APPLY CONDITIONER TO YOUR ROOTS. It will weigh down your hair.

- SLACK OFF WHEN RINSING A MOISTURIZING HAIR MASK OUT OF YOUR HAIR and off your scalp, or the residue will make your hair look and feel greasy.

- TRY TO BRUSH YOUR CURLS. Even using a spiral brush, you will lose the shape and bring on frizz.

- APPLY SHINE SERUM TO THE FRONT OF YOUR HAIR FIRST, like the sides or top of your head. "Since the most product distributes in the spot where you first apply it, start in the back, with most of your hair, and then work your way toward your face," explains Hershberger. Otherwise you end up with too much product on too little hair.

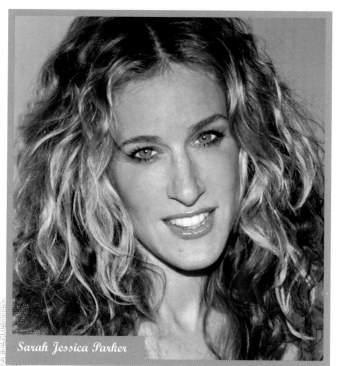

Sarah Jessica Parker

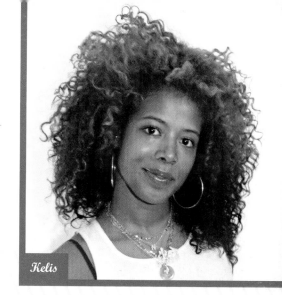

Kelis

TIGHT CURLS

YOU HAVE TIGHT CURLY HAIR IF . . .

*Your tresses are a beautiful mass of tight curls and coils.

*You use a comb or pick to style your hair rather than a brush.

*You only have to wash your hair once a week, if that. It doesn't get greasy very often.

TIGHT CURLY HAIR DOS

- "CUT YOUR HAIR AFTER IT'S BEEN BLOW-DRIED AS STRAIGHT AS POSSIBLE SO THE CUT IS EVEN," says celebrity hair stylist Oscar James, who works on stars including Halle Berry, Tyra Banks, and Jada Pinkett Smith. Face-framing long layers look great if you have a heart-shaped, square, or round face. For a square face, long bangs look great.

- TREAT YOURSELF TO A TRIM EVERY TWO-AND-A-HALF MONTHS, to keep your hair healthy and neat looking.

- "WASH HAIR EVERY ONE TO TWO WEEKS WITH A MOISTUR-IZING SHAMPOO," advises James. If you wash your hair too much, it can become dry and your scalp may get itchy and irritated.

- CONDITION HAIR EVERY TIME YOU SUDS UP with a moisturizing conditioner or hot oil to keep tresses soft and shiny.

- BRING OUT YOUR NATURAL TEXTURE WITH LIGHTWEIGHT STYLING PRODUCTS, like mousses and serums, which will coat your hair shaft and fight frizz without weighing down hair.

- "MAKE HAIR GLISTEN WITH A SILICON SERUM. Apply it from just below the roots to tips of dry hair," says James.

TIGHT CURLY HAIR DON'TS

- CUT HAIR WHEN IT IS CURLY—wet or dry—because it is hard to create an even shape, says James. When hair is dried straight, "you can see exactly what you are getting," he adds.

- OVERWASH YOUR HAIR. It can dry out.

- "USE GEL-BASED PRODUCTS TO STYLE HAIR or it will become crunchy and stiff," says James.

- GREASE YOUR SCALP WITH HEAVY POMADES OR CREAMS, which can clog hair follicles.

CHEMICALLY RELAXED HAIR

YOU HAVE CHEMICALLY RELAXED HAIR IF (and you probably know this already) . . .

*You have had your hair chemically relaxed in a salon or with an at-home kit.

*Your hair naturally dries less curly than it did before it was relaxed.

*Your hair is on the dry side, plus it breaks and tangles easily.

CHEMICALLY RELAXED HAIR DOS

- "CUT CHEMICALLY RELAXED HAIR AFTER IT HAS BEEN BLOW-DRIED STRAIGHT for the most even shape, about every two-and-a-half months," says James.

- USE A RAZOR TO CUT HAIR TO CREATE A SOFT PIECE-Y LOOK if you have a square-, oval-, or heart-shaped face, or scissors to cut hair to create a more blunt, even style if you have a round face.

- WASH EVERY ONE TO TWO WEEKS WITH A MOISTURIZING SHAMPOO. Rinse thoroughly so you leave no residue on your scalp, which can make it become itchy.

- CONDITION YOUR HAIR WITH A RINSE-OUT OR LEAVE-IN CONDITIONER EVERY TIME YOU WASH. For the healthiest hair, alternate between the rinse-out and leave-in variety every three times you wash. To be sure that you have conditioned your entire head of hair evenly, "comb through conditioner with a wide-toothed comb," adds James.

- HAVE FUN AND CREATE A NEW TEXTURE IN YOUR HAIR. First, apply a setting lotion from roots to tips of damp strands; then twist or braid sections of your hair; blow-dry with a diffuser.

- TREAT YOURSELF TO MOISTURIZING CONDITIONING TREATMENT IN A SALON OR AT HOME ONCE A MONTH. In a salon, they will pump up the power of a moisturizing conditioner with heat. At home, after you have applied a deep conditioner to your damp strands, cover your hair with a shower cap and top with a towel that you have warmed in the dryer. The towel will warm up your hair so the conditioner works even better.

- WEAR A SILK SCARF AT NIGHT TO PROTECT HAIR FROM BREAKING, when it rubs against your pillowcase.

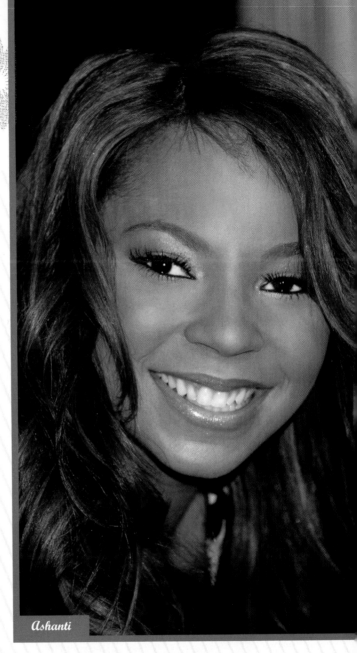

Ashanti

CHEMICALLY RELAXED HAIR DON'TS

- CUT YOUR HAIR WHEN IT IS WET. You might end up with an uneven style, since hair is only stick-straight when it is blow-dried that way.

- WEIGH DOWN YOUR HAIR WITH HEAVY WAXES AND OILS. They won't make hair more shiny and manageable, just greasy.

- "OVERSTYLE YOUR HAIR by using a hair-dryer or straightening iron every single day, or your hair can become brittle," says James.

- SHAMPOO YOUR HAIR OR MASSAGE YOUR SCALP THE SAME DAY YOU ARE GOING TO RELAX YOUR STRANDS, because your scalp may become irritated.

THE HAIR HEALTH TEST

*O*K, before you can figure out what to do with your hair, you need to find out what shape it's in. Below are three little tests that will help you to determine whether your hair has split ends, is too dry, or is just plain frazzled. Try them all and then read on for all the info and advice you'll ever need to get your best hair ever.

1. Pull out one strand of your hair. Grab it between your thumb and index finger on each hand, holding it fairly taut. Now pull it apart a bit more. If it snaps immediately your hair may be too dry. If it stretches a little bit and then bounces back to its original shape when you stop pulling, your hair is pretty healthy. If it stretches a bit but doesn't bounce back into its original shape, it's a little dry and damaged, but not beyond repair.

2. Pull out one strand of your hair. Fill a glass with water and drop the hair into it. If the strand sinks to the bottom, that means your locks are parched. Why? A regular strand floats on top because it's fully hydrated, therefore it can't absorb any more moisture. A sinking strand is so dry that it drinks up H_2O from the glass.

3. Pull out one strand of your hair (last one, we swear). Grab a sewing needle and try to thread the strand through the eye (the end, not the root part of the hair). If it threads through no problem, your hair is in great shape. If it gets snagged, that means the hair cuticle is damaged and frayed, or you have split ends, making it difficult to fit through the eye of the needle.

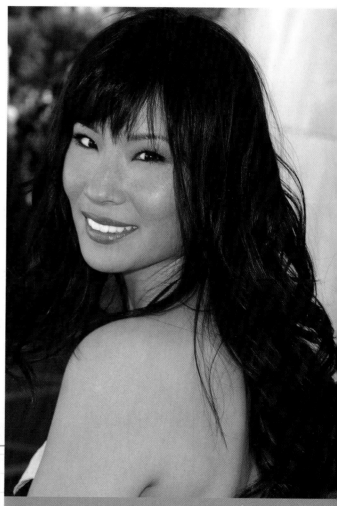

Want to know Lucy's healthy hair secret? Turn to "Star Treatments" on page 28 for her stylist's tips.

What now? Well, the point here is to show you that no one's hair is perfect. The next chapter is chock-full of ideas for making your hair look fabulous. Everyone has the ability to have great hair. All you need is some professional advice, the right products, and a few Hollywood insider tips on how the stars keep their strands looking fantastic.

WHAT'S YOUR DAMAGE?

*H*air is pretty fragile stuff, and if you spend time coloring it, blasting it with a blow-dryer or generally ignoring it, eventually it will end up looking less than luscious. While you can't totally repair most of these mane mishaps, you can at least make them look less obvious as well as prevent future foul-ups. Leanne Citrone of the Chris McMillan Salon in Beverly Hills (who has pampered such heads as Lauren Ambrose) tells you how to avoid hair horrors, as well as how to hide any current damage while your mane gets pampered back to perfect!

THE DAMAGE: SPLIT ENDS

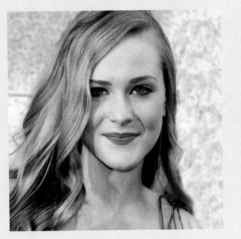

Keep long hair like Evan Rachel Wood's healthy and split-free with timely trims.

HOW IT HAPPENS: When hair doesn't get regular trims, the ends of the hair shaft will get weak and split. Also, if your hair is really dried out, you'll end up with frayed bottoms because what few natural oils do come out of the hair follicle never make it down that far.

HOW TO AVOID: See your stylist. If you're trying to grow your hair and don't want to get a trim, think again. Once hair starts to split, it won't stop. It just keeps splitting farther and farther up the hair shaft, meaning you'll have to cut way more off than if you'd kept up with your regular hair appointment. Finally, don't let your 'do dry out. Make sure you use a good conditioner appropriate for your hair type every time you are in the shower.

HOW TO HIDE IT QUICKLY: If your ends are a total splitfest, you need to use a styling product to add texture. The best remedy is to take a small amount of pomade or wax (the size of a pea is perfect) and rub it between your hands before gently applying it to the bottom two inches of your strands.

THE DAMAGE: FRIED STRANDS

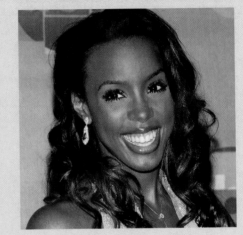

If you love to show off hairstyles tht require a lot of heat like Kelly Rowland, make sure to get a good conditioner.

HOW IT HAPPENS: When hair is bombarded with too many heat stylers (straightening irons and blow-dryers), the hair shaft gets dried out, making hair look dry and frizzy.

HOW TO AVOID: Keep your locks from drying out by shampooing every other day and only applying it at the roots, which are always the greasiest. Apply conditioner every day, and once a week use a deep-conditioning cream on your strands. Let it soak in for half an hour (perfect to do if you're taking a bath). Finally, before blow-drying or straightening, make sure your hair is about 80 percent dry so you don't need to have heat on it for too long. Also, always coat hair with spray designed to protect hair from heat styling before drying.

HOW TO HIDE IT QUICKLY: While you can't totally fix fried hair in five minutes, you can fake healthy hair by applying shine-enhancing products like serums and sprays—thicker hair should choose the serums, fine hair the sprays.

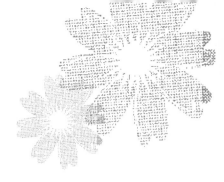

THE DAMAGE: A DULL 'DO

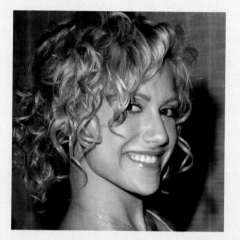

Heavily styled strands like Brittany Murphy's need a good clarifying shampoo.

HOW IT HAPPENS: When hair isn't healthy, the first thing to go is the shine. This is caused by everything from excessive heat styling to coloring to product buildup.

HOW TO AVOID: As well as keeping hair healthy with lots of conditioning treatments, it's a good idea to use a clarifying shampoo once a week, especially if you use a lot of styling products. Clarifying shampoos work by stripping away dull-enhancing ingredients that build up over time when you use styling products (waxes and pomades are the key buildup culprits because they are the greasiest). Also, minerals found in our everyday water can get stuck in your strands and tone down your natural shine. Finally, if you love to flat-iron or blow-dry your hair often, start spritzing it with a leave-in conditioner before styling—this will protect your hair and help it to remain healthy.

HOW TO HIDE IT QUICKLY: If your hair has lost its luster, try a shine-enhancing product with light-reflecting ingredients. For fine hair, look for a shine spray that you lightly mist over the head. Thicker hair can handle something a little heavier, such as a serum. Remember, when applying shine-enhancing products, apply a little at a time—too much at once will just make hair look greasy.

THE DAMAGE: BRASSY COLOR

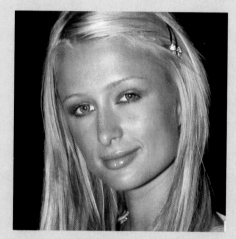

If you're going to take your color to the extreme, like Paris Hilton, make sure you pamper it too.

HOW IT HAPPENS: You've tinted your tresses and now they're looking either faded, or, if you've gone blond, a bit yellow.

HOW TO AVOID: Let a professional take over. If you're coloring your hair at home with a permanent dye or bleach, it's tough to make your hair look as fab as when a pro does it. When you add color to your hair, the hair shaft is "opened up" and the color is "deposited." However, just like your favorite pair of jeans fade after tons of washes, so does your hair (for more on dyeing your hair, go to "Color-Coded" on page 110). When you have your hair colored at a salon, they can apply a glossing treatment after the color product (it's like a mega-conditioner that makes your hair super shiny) so your hair will hold the color longer. Also, ask them what products they recommend to help your hair keep its color once you get home.

HOW TO HIDE IT QUICKLY: Hair that looks brassy is often dull, so using a shine-enhancing gel or silicone serum when styling will help. Also, there are a ton of shampoos and conditioners on the market for color-treated hair that work by depositing a little bit of color every time you lather up so your color really holds up.

DON'T TYPECAST YOUR HAIR

*N*eed a couple of ideas about what to do with your 'do? Well, no one is more versatile with their tresses than celebrities. Not only do they go to more parties and events than the rest of us (perfect excuse to get busy with the blow-dryer), but they also use the best Hollywood stylists to get them glam. Here are some styles that some of our favorite celebrities have stepped out in recently. If there's one you love, take the picture with you next time you get your hair cut.

SHORT...Just because you've got a close crop doesn't mean you can't switch it up and get creative.

ALYSSA MILANO shows that hair can be super short and still look super chic.

Even a cut as close as **FANTASIA BARRINO**'s can look glam by spiking up the top and piecing up the bangs.

When **KEIRA KNIGHTLEY** chopped off her long locks, her look instantly became edgier.

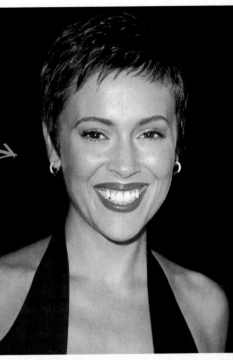

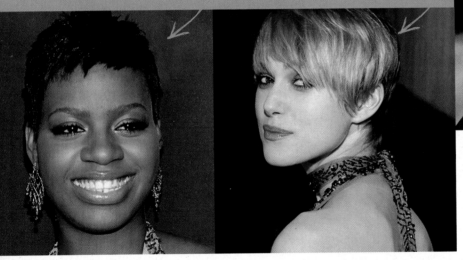

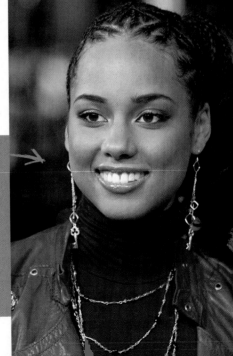

BRAIDS...Add a personalized touch to your cornrows by twisting, crisscrossing, and curling them up.

With her intricately designed braids and high ponytail, **ALICIA KEYS** shows the perfect way to funk up a classic updo.

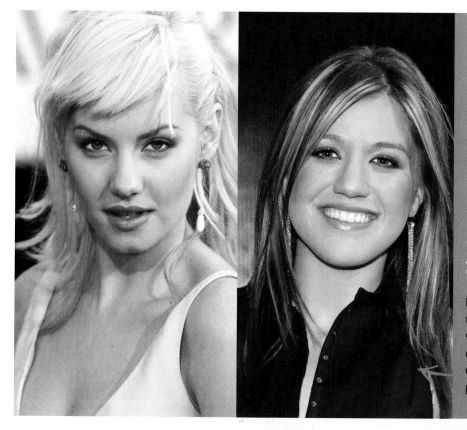

MEDIUM...
Anything goes with a mane that's a little in-between. Up or down, you're good to go.

ELISHA CUTHBERT's shoulder-skimming style looks low maintenance and chic when it's clipped back.

Chunky blond streaks give **KELLY CLARKSON'S** shoulder-length 'do pizzazz.

LONG...Whether curly or straight, lengthy locks always look lovely.

JESSICA SIMPSON's soft waves are created by putting hair in curlers before blow-drying.

SUCHIN PAK makes long hair funky with blunt bangs, chunky face-framing layers, and a hint of pink.

JENNIFER FREEMAN's flowing curls are tangled and tousled beautifully.

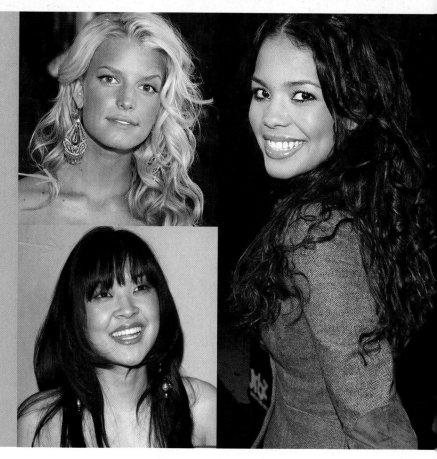

OUR TOP 10 HAIRSTYLES

There are some stars whose style we just can't get enough of—especially when it comes to hair. And while many celebs change their hair constantly, some of them manage to look fabulous whatever look they choose. Check out our picks for best red-carpet ready haircuts as well as tips on how to style these looks so you can road test the tresses of your favorite celebs.

1. VaVa Volume

Why We Love It

Jessica is a total girlie girl and her hair shows that. It's a simple cut that goes a few inches below the shoulders, with longish bangs that Jessica always sweeps to the side. There are layers around her face as well as layers all around the bottom half of her hair to create volume. This 'do, created by her mane guy, Ken Pavés, is casual as well as totally feminine thanks to some loose waves.

What You'll Need

- ❏ VOLUMIZING SPRAY
- ❏ BLOW-DRYER WITH BOTH HOT AND COOL SETTINGS
- ❏ 8–12 LARGE VELCRO ROLLERS
- ❏ LARGE BOBBY PINS
- ❏ MEDIUM-HOLD HAIRSPRAY
- ❏ ROUND BRUSH

How To Get The Look

1. Spritz damp hair with volumizing spray from the roots all the way down to the ends (this is most easily done by holding up sections of hair from the head and spraying section by section). Next, flip hair over so it's all hanging down and blow-dry until hair is almost dry.

2. Using the Velcro rollers, roll small sections of hair beginning at the front and center of your head. Attach with a pin to keep the roller in place. The next roller should sit right behind roller #1. Run a row of rollers back to the nape of your neck. When you've completed the center row, do a row on either side of the center row arcing back over the crown of your head.

3. Let hair set for 20 minutes and then give each section a blast with the blow-dryer until hair feels dry. Switch the blow-dryer to the cool setting and blast again. "The cool air really helps to lock in the curl by sealing down the cuticle on the hair shaft," says Hollywood hair guy Campbell McAuley, who has worked with Lindsay Lohan.

4. Remove the rollers, part hair on the side, and give hair a light brush. Spritz with medium-hold hairspray to keep curls in place.

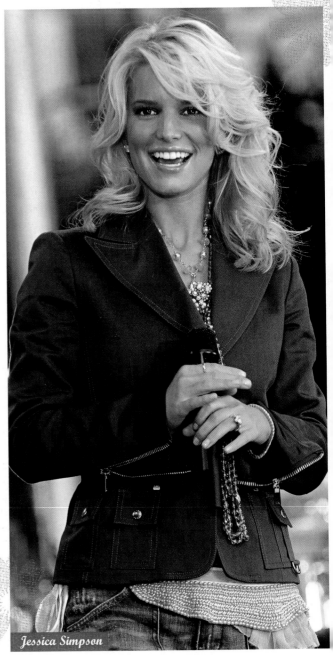

Jessica Simpson

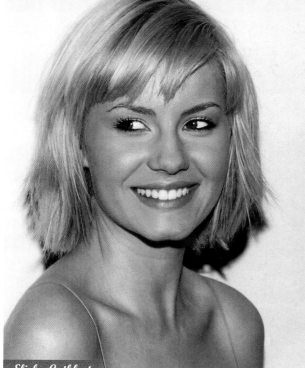

Elisha Cuthbert

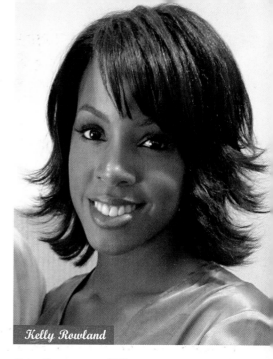

Kelly Rowland

2. Edgy Bob

Why We Love It

Elisha Cuthbert makes the bob look totally funky and fresh. This just-below-the-chin cut with thick bangs is given a new spin by cutting a few long layers around the bottom. "Elisha's hair also gets great movement because it's colored," says hairstylist Gabriel Georgiou, who has worked with the star. Dyed strands look a bit thicker because the hair color puffs out the hair cuticle so it's actually a volumizing trick for any girl with fine hair.

What You'll Need
❏ VOLUMIZING GEL
❏ VOLUMIZING SPRAY
❏ POMADE
❏ BLOW-DRYER
❏ ROUND BRUSH

How To Get The Look

1. Apply a quarter-sized dollop of gel to damp hair, starting at the roots and working your way down the hair shaft.

2. Spritz a volumizing spray only at the roots, where you need a little lift. Blow-dry hair by grabbing a one-inch-square section from the nape of your neck and placing the brush on the underside of the section close to the roots. Point the nozzle of the blow-dryer in a downward direction, above the brush. Slowly pull the brush down toward the ends, moving the blow-dryer in the same direction at the same time, which gives you a nice straight look. Do the whole head like this until it's dry.

3. Part hair on the side and then rub a pea-size amount of pomade on the palm of your hands. Distribute the pomade to the ends of the hair.

4. Add a little pomade to bangs to keep them in place.

3. Feminine Flip

Why We Love It

Kelly's shoulder-length style needs to be totally versatile since this singer goes from one glam event to the next. This shoulder-length flip can morph into so many styles because of the thick eyebrow-length bangs, as well as the shorter layers around the face. There are also longer layers throughout the rest of the hair to give it movement. "Kelly likes to change her hair a lot and is always willing to try a new trend," says Kimberly Kimble, who has worked with the girls of Destiny's Child as well as Gabrielle Union.

What You'll Need
❏ SHINE SPRAY
❏ STRAIGHTENING IRON
❏ CURLING IRON
❏ SHINE SERUM

How To Get The Look

1. Start with freshly blow- or air-dried hair.

2. Spritz hair all over with the shine spray. "I always spray this on beforehand to protect the hair from heat styling," recommends Kimble.

3. Take the straightening iron and grab a one-inch-square section of hair. Clamp the straightening iron down right at the roots and quickly run it down the length of the hair shaft to the ends (don't let the iron linger on any section of the hair or it could fry your strands). When you have straightened the whole head, take small sections around the face and flip them up using the curling iron—you don't have to roll up the hair all the way to the roots, just stop about halfway.

4. To finish off this style, pour a little shine serum into the palm of your hand and use it to smooth down bangs and any pesky flyaways.

4. Loose Curls

Why We Love It

This is the perfect soft wavy look. Reaching almost to her waist, Stone's thick, naturally wavy strands have some long layers cut into them to enhance the curl. "Joss has amazing hair and because it's thick, she can get away with wearing it this long without it looking too fine," says hairstylist Cheryl Marks, who has worked on another curly girl, Sarah Jessica Parker.

What You'll Need

☐ LEAVE-IN CONDITIONER SPRAY
☐ VOLUMIZING SPRAY
☐ BLOW-DRYER
☐ CURLING IRON
☐ STYLING WAX

How To Get The Look

1. Spritz a leave-in conditioner spray on damp ends to keep them from drying out.

2. Spritz a volumizing spray only at the roots, where you need a little lift. Blow-dry hair by flipping your head over.

3. When hair is almost dry, don't brush it too smooth; instead, use the curling iron to add some extra waves. Take a one-inch-square section of hair and, starting at the ends, roll the section up around the barrel of the curling iron (don't roll up the hair all the way to the roots; stop about halfway).

4. When you've finished curling, apply a touch of wax to your hands and style hair with your fingers to make the ends look cool and piece-y.

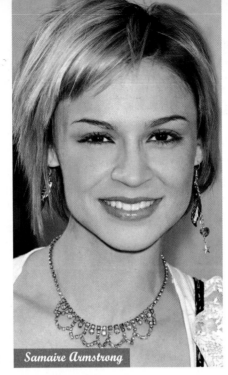

Samaire Armstrong

5. Short and Choppy

Why We Love It

This perfectly edgy cut that works so many ways. Samaire's fine hair is cut into a jagged chin-length bob that is cut shorter in the back than the front, with a few layers around the face and choppy, super-short bangs. "Adding a lot of layers to a style like this means that it can either look spiky and messy or smooth and pretty," says McAuley.

What You'll Need

☐ LIGHT-HOLD GEL
☐ BLOW-DRYER
☐ PADDLE BRUSH
☐ LIGHT STYLING WAX

How To Get The Look

1. Apply a quarter-sized dollop of gel from roots to ends on damp hair.

2. Blow-dry hair while mussing it up with your fingers as you go—this style is not about looking neat.

3. When hair is dry, part on the side and smooth out with the brush.

4. Apply a pea-sized amount of wax on your hands and smooth it over the hair before using your hands to give a little volume lift at the roots.

6. Lightly Layered

Why We Love It

This chic, simple straight style has a bit of rocker edge thanks to some long, choppy layers. "Nicky's hair is medium thick and in great condition," says Brant Mayfield, who has worked on the dark-haired party girl (who has some of the shiniest strands around). Her below-the-shoulders cut is easily copied by adding a couple of longish layers around the face. This cut will work on all hair types, even curly hair.

What You'll Need

☐ VOLUMIZING SPRAY
☐ BLOW-DRYER
☐ ROUND BRUSH
☐ SHINE SPRAY

How To Get The Look

1. Spritz a volumizing spray on damp roots, where you need a little lift. To do this, grab a section of hair, pull it up, and spray right at the roots.

2. To blow-dry hair, grab a one-inch-square section from the nape of your neck and place the brush on the underside of the section close to the roots. Point the nozzle of the blow-dryer in a downward direction, above the brush. Slowly pull the brush down toward the ends, moving the blow-dryer in the same direction at the same time.

3. When hair is dry, lightly spritz with shine spray and muss it up with your fingers. "This style shouldn't look too groomed," adds Mayfield.

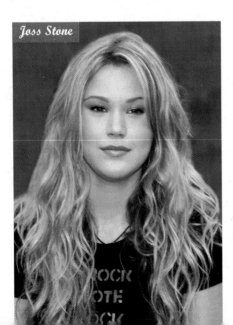

Joss Stone

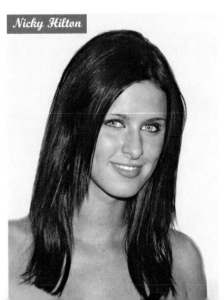

Nicky Hilton

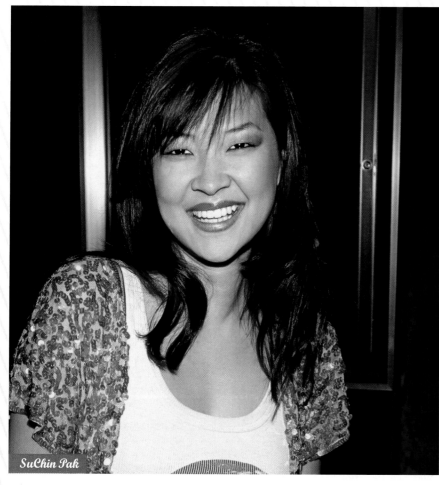

SuChin Pak

8. Perfect Curls

Why We Love It

This style is a perfect example of how pretty curly hair can look when it's left natural. Hilarie's hair falls just above the shoulder but has lots of layers in it to thin out the curls and keep her hair from looking puffy. "The less you do to style curly hair, the better it looks," says Colleen Conway, who has styled Jessica Alba's strands.

What You'll Need

❑ CURL-ENHANCING GEL
❑ BLOW-DRYER
❑ SHINE SPRAY

How To Get The Look

1. Start with damp hair and apply gel to roots only, about an inch up the hair shaft.

2. Lift up sections of hair and point the blow-dryer right at the roots (this gives you the same great lift that Hilarie has at the top of her head).

3. Blow-dry the rest of the hair but stop before it's totally dry (if you get it too dry it will frizz). "Curly hair always looks best if it's allowed to dry naturally," adds Conway.

4. Take curls and wrap them around your index finger, holding them for a few seconds before letting them go—this helps to define the curl.

5. When you're done, spritz strands with the shine spray to enhance gloss.

7. Flattering Fringe

Why We Love It

This is a great long hairstyle for girls with lots of hair since it creates definition with lots of layered curls or waves. "Asian hair is often very thick and very straight," says Robert Hallowell, who is Lucy Liu's mane guy. The red highlights around SuChin's face give this simple style a cool edge.

What You'll Need

❑ MEDIUM-HOLD GEL
❑ BLOW-DRYER
❑ ROUND BRUSH
❑ CURLING IRON
❑ HAIRSPRAY

How To Get The Look

1. Start with damp hair and apply a quarter-sized dollop of gel from roots to ends.

2. Blow-dry hair by grabbing a one-inch-square section from the nape of your neck and placing the brush on the underside of the section close to the roots. Point the nozzle of the blow-dryer in a downward direction, above the brush. Slowly pull the brush down toward the ends, moving the blow-dryer in the same direction at the same time.

3. When hair is dry, take the curling iron and curl the front sections in a forward direction around the face. "It's always flattering to have the hair frame the face," adds Hallowell.

4. Lightly spritz your whole head with hairspray to help your style last.

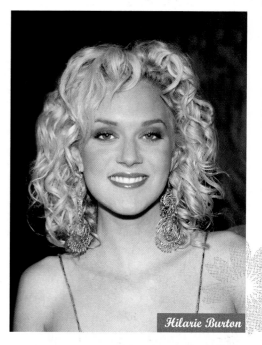

Hilarie Burton

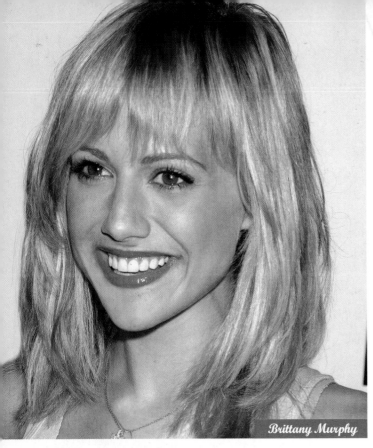
Brittany Murphy

9. Sexy Shag

Why We Love It

While her natural color is medium brown, Brittany Murphy likes to add highlights to her strands to turn them golden blond. Add a just-past-the-shoulders cut with lots of layers and eyebrow-skimming bangs and you've got one great hairstyle. "Bangs are a great way to add personality to a long hairstyle," says John Francis, Hollywood hairstylist who has worked with Courteney Cox Arquette.

What You'll Need

- ❑ VOLUMIZING SPRAY
- ❑ BLOW-DRYER
- ❑ ROUND BRUSH
- ❑ STRAIGHTENING IRON
- ❑ SHINE SPRAY

How To Get The Look

1. Start by spritzing a volumizing spray on damp roots, where you need a little lift. "If you spray a volumizing spray all over your head, it will make hair too heavy and just weigh it down," says Francis.

2. To blow-dry hair, grab a one-inch-square section from the nape of your neck and place the brush on the underside of the section close to the roots. Point the nozzle of the blow-dryer in a downward direction, above the brush. Slowly pull the brush down toward the ends, moving the blow-dryer in the same direction at the same time.

3. Take the straightening iron and clamp it on the ends of the hair (about 1 or 2 inches from the bottom), to help them lie smooth.

4. Spritz your whole head lightly with a shine spray to add some megawatt superstar gloss.

10. Hot Rocker

Why We Love It

Ashlee's long locks get a rock and roll twist thanks to thick, eyebrow-skimming bangs and long layers. "Having layers like Ashlee's gives you a ton of options when it comes to styling," says Hollywood stylist Cheryl Marks who has styled Cameron Diaz. "It's easy to add curl, but it looks equally cool stick-straight."

What You'll Need:

- ❑ VOLUMIZING SPRAY
- ❑ WIDE-TOOTHED COMB
- ❑ BLOW-DRYER
- ❑ ROUND BRUSH
- ❑ LARGE-BARRELED CURLING IRON
- ❑ SHINE SPRAY

How To Get The Look

1. Spritz damp hair with volumizing spray from the roots all the way down to the ends (this is most easily done by holding up sections of hair from the head and spraying section by section). Comb hair to get rid of any tangles.

2. To blow-dry hair, by grab a one-inch-square section from the nape of your neck and place the brush on the underside of the section, close to the roots. Point the nozzle of the blow-dryer in a downward direction, above the brush. Slowly pull the brush down toward the ends, moving the blow-dryer in the same direction at the same time.

3. When hair is dry, take the curling iron and wrap sections of hair around the barrel. Don't leave the curling iron on for too long (five seconds is fine) and focus on curling the front section of your hair.

4. When you have enough curls, don't brush them; instead, just arrange hair using your fingers. Spritz with shine spray.

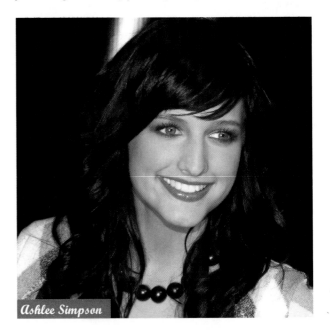
Ashlee Simpson

10 TIPS TO BEING A SALON DIVA

*H*ave you ever left a hair salon with a haircut you didn't like? Did you ask for a trim and the stylist hacked off five inches? The trick is being able to communicate with the person cutting or coloring your hair. We asked Nelson Chan at the Estetica Salon in Beverly Hills (who is Sarah Michelle Gellar's colorist) for the inside scoop on getting what you want, the right questions to ask, and how to navigate the whole salon experience.

1. If there's a certain cut you have in mind, always go armed with pictures. Your idea of a Jennifer Aniston haircut may be totally different from your stylist's. With pics in hand, you're guaranteed to end up on the same page.

2. The same goes for color. Bring in pics of the shade you want. Many colorists say that one of the main hurdles when choosing a color for a client is when a client has unrealistic expectations. Just because Christina Aguilera goes from one extreme to the next with her dye job doesn't mean that it will work for you, so pics will help you and your colorist make a realistic selection.

3. When discussing your cut or color with your hairstylist, make sure to tell him or her how much time you are willing to spend doing your hair in the morning and what kind of lifestyle you lead. If you're a wash 'n' go girl who plays soccer every day, a style that needs lots of blow-drying and products may not be right for you.

4. Always show up 10 minutes early to your appointment so you have enough time to chat with the stylist before she begins working on your hair.

5. Pay attention while the stylist is cutting your hair, so you can stop her if she's doing something you don't like. A lot of girls bury their heads in magazines until the stylist is finished and then are bummed out when they don't like the results.

6. Speaking of bummed about the results, if you hate your new cut it's best to tell your stylist while you are still at the salon, instead of going home and bursting into tears. You don't have to rant and rave, just say something like "this is not really what I had in mind." Good stylists want you to be happy, so they'll try to fix it if possible.

7. Don't wash your hair the day of your appointment. Colorists say it's much better to color hair that's a little bit greasy because the natural oils protect your scalp (this is key if you're considering bleach, because it can sting).

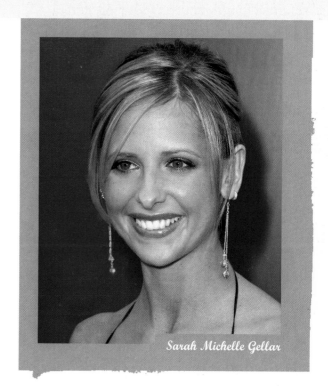
Sarah Michelle Gellar

8. Ask the stylist what kind of products she recommends for your hair. This goes for shampoo, conditioner, and styling stuff. Even though they probably sell products at their salon, don't feel obligated to buy them; but if your stylist suggests a gel and you've always used a mousse, take note.

9. Ask your stylist for advice on how to take care of your hair once you are home. Ask how often you should shampoo, if you need a deep conditioning, and when to come back for your next appointment.

10. Figuring out how to tip can be a bit tricky, but here are the basic rules: If your stylist owns the salon, you don't have to tip him or her. Otherwise, give him or her 15 to 20 percent of the total price of your haircut or color. Also, don't forget to tip the person who shampoos your hair a couple of dollars.

HAIR 911: YOUR WORST STRAND SNAFUS SOLVED

Who doesn't have hair horror every once in a while? Whether it's wrangling some stubborn knots or finding the perfect prom style, we've got you covered by rounding up the answers to some of your worst 'do dilemmas. Hair guru Crystal Tesinsky, who has worked with Zooey Deschanel and Nicole Richie, and stylist Cheryl Marks, who has tamed the tresses of Cameron Diaz, show you how to handle your hair.

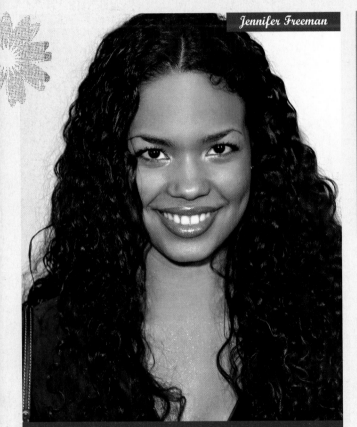

Jennifer Freeman

Q. My hair is tangle central, especially at the back of my neck. Every day I have to wrestle with a brush to get them out. What gives?

A. It's common to have strand snags at the back of the neck, since a lot of the time they're caused by your hair rubbing against the collar of your shirt or sweater. "The best place to take care of tangles is in the shower," says Tesinsky. Before you shower, brush hair thoroughly, starting at the ends and working your way up to the roots. Once in the shower, wash and condition your hair, and use a wide-toothed comb to work conditioner through your hair before rinsing it out. Finally, when you hop out of the shower, don't rub or twist your hair up in a towel to dry it, as this can cause new knots. Instead, blot hair with a towel until it feels damp, comb it through again, and let it air-dry.

Q. I cut my own bangs and now they look horrible. Is there anything I can do?

A. Well, there is no way to make your hair grow faster than it already does (half an inch per month is average), so if your fringe is super-short the only way to cover up your botched cut is with styling products and hair accessories. When hair is damp, apply some strong-hold gel and blow-dry bangs off to the side. You do this by brushing them sideways while pointing the dryer in the direction you want the hair to go. Also, never underestimate the power of a cute clip. If you trimmed your bangs and made them look uneven, however, hightail it to your stylist. By the way, most stylists offer free bang trims between haircuts so there's really no need for you to snip your own strands.

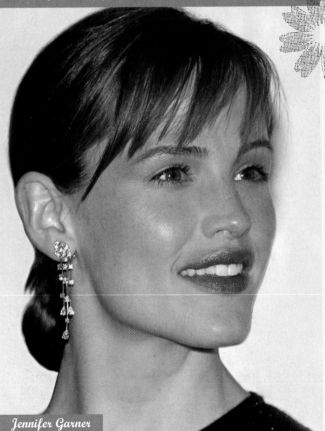

Jennifer Garner

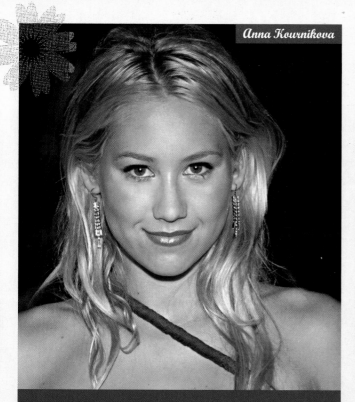

Anna Kournikova

Q. I play sports most days after school, so I often end up shampooing twice a day. Is this OK or am I damaging my hair?

A. While you're not doing serious damage, you probably are overcleaning it. "Your hair doesn't need to be shampooed every day, let alone twice a day," says Marks. "You can get your hair clean without lathering up all the time." If you have to shower in the morning, just scrub your scalp using your fingers while the water washes over it, as this will rinse out some of the scalp oils naturally. After practice, if you feel you have to lather up, make sure to use a gentle shampoo that is specifically meant to be used every day. On days when you don't play sports, try to skip lathering up. "If you think your hair looks greasy, just give it a good brush, as this helps to distribute the natural oils down the hair shaft, as opposed to them just collecting up at the roots," says Marks.

Q: I'd love to wear my hair up for prom, but I want something simple that's not going to fall apart after a couple of hours on the dance floor. Any ideas?

A: "The easiest updo is a chic low ponytail," says Tesinsky. To make a pony look a little dressier, start by parting hair on the side (a pony always looks more chic with a part instead of just brushed straight back). Secure hair with an elastic band at the nape of the neck (at the bottom in the middle) and conceal the band by taking a small section of hair from the ponytail, wrapping it around the elastic and tucking in the ends underneath. "If you want to add some extra sparkle, you can also clip a rhinestone barrette in the back, right next to the ponytail."

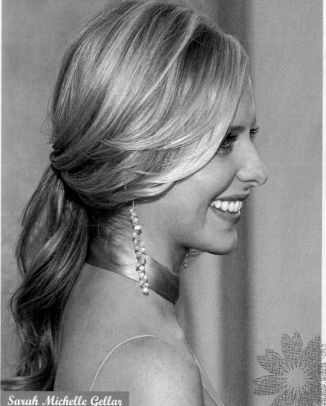

Sarah Michelle Gellar

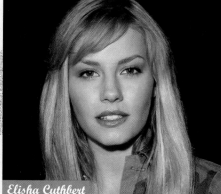

Elisha Cuthbert

Q. I have blond hair and every summer it turns green from the chlorine in the pool. Is there anything I can do to avoid Kermit hair?

A. "Chlorine contains bleach and an ingredient called algaecide, both of which contribute to lime-colored locks," says Marks. To avoid green hair, always soak hair with regular water before hopping in the pool—that way it soaks up moisture from the natural water as opposed to the chlorinated H_2O. When you get out of the pool, rinse it again with regular water to wash out any pool residue. Also, after a pool party, wash your hair with a clarifying shampoo, which works to wash away any chemical or product residues that are left on the hair. Since clarifying shampoos can be drying, only lather up with them once or twice a week.

COLOR-CODED: WHICH DIVA'S DYE JOB IS RIGHT FOR YOU?

CHANGING HAIR COLOR IS ONE WAY STARS STAY IN THE SPOTLIGHT. WHEN IT COMES TO HAIR COLOR THERE ARE TONS OF FORMULATIONS AND PRODUCTS TO CHOOSE FROM. DO YOU WANT SOMETHING THAT WILL WASH OUT QUICKLY OR STAY PUT FOR MONTHS? COLORIST LUCIE DOUGHTY (WHO HAS WORKED ON JENNIFER LOVE HEWITT) GAVE US THE LOWDOWN ON ALL THE DIFFERENT TREATMENTS AND TRICKS FOR COLORING YOUR TRESSES.

HIGHLIGHTS

WHAT IT IS: This involves having small sections of your hair permanently dyed a few shades lighter than your natural shade.

WHAT IT CAN DO FOR YOU: These are great if you want to change your color a little bit. Also, highlights can be really flattering, especially getting a few around the face, since it can help to lighten your look (think sun-kissed).

WHO SHOULD TRY IT: Anyone who wants a subtle change that doesn't require a lot of upkeep. Since highlights don't cover your whole head, the new growth isn't that visible right away and you can go a while between color appointments (three to four months). Also, if you chemically straighten your hair and it's already a little fragile, highlights are the way to go, since they are not as damaging as dyeing your whole head.

GET INSPIRED BY:

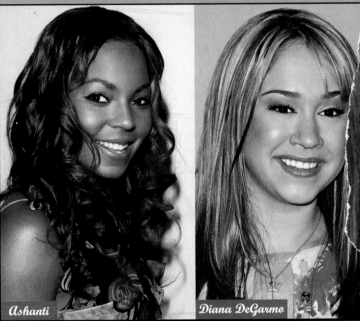

Ashanti   *Diana DeGarmo*

SEMI-PERMANENT COLOR

WHAT IT IS: This is like a color rinse for your hair. It has no bleach in it, so it can't lighten your hair; it only makes it a few shades darker or subtly different. The results last for about six to eight shampoos.

WHAT IT CAN DO FOR YOU: It's great if you feel like your natural hue is a bit blah. For example, if you're a brunette babe, try a red semi-permanent to warm up your existing shade. Or an ash blonde can try a golden semi-permanent for subtle sparkle. It's also very good for making your existing shade look a bit shinier.

WHO SHOULD TRY IT: This is great if you're the type of girl who doesn't want to take the plunge with a permanent, long-lasting color. Also, if you've never colored you hair before, this is a great way to start because the change isn't too drastic and the shade washes out pretty quickly if you don't like it.

GET INSPIRED BY:

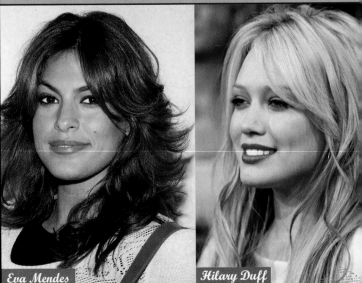

Eva Mendes   *Hilary Duff*

Serena Williams

Judging by her morphing mane, we think this athlete is an ace on the court as well as on the red carpet. Her secret for making every hair shade work for her is to always pick warm colors that complement her skin tone.

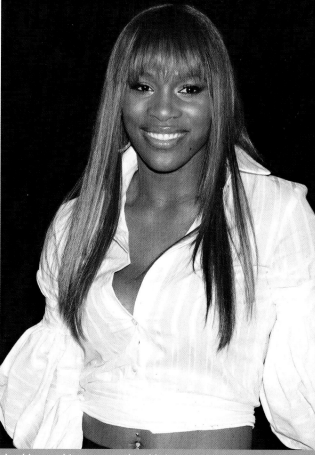

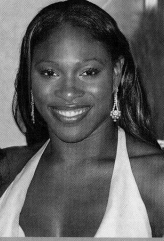

Her natural chocolate hue with some serious shine to boot

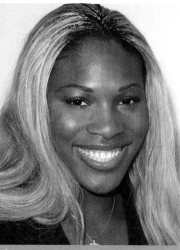

Going for the gold look

Looking cool in copper-colored hair extensions

Pink

While she's ditched the fluorescent hue that she was named after, this singer still keeps us guessing with her hair color. While her dye ideas aren't for everyone, she can pull them off because she has such a fierce attitude and style.

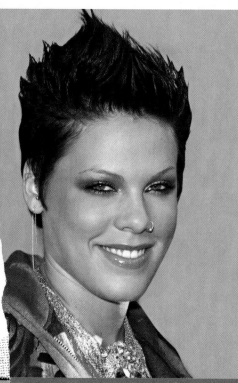

This midnight shade looks dramatic and seriously edgy.

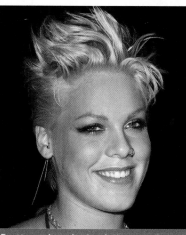

Pretty and punky in platinum spikes

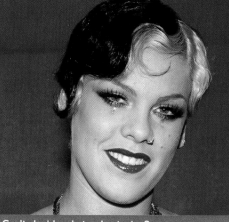

Can't decide what color to try? How about both!

HOLLYWOOD'S TOP STYLISTS TELL ALL

*W*ho doesn't wonder how the stars always keep their strands looking so good. We ask Ruby Weifer (who has worked with Mischa Barton), Mark Slicker (who counts Amanda Bynes as one of his fans), and Crystal Tesinsky (the strand styler for Laura Prepon and Nicole Richie). With all of this star-studded strand power, we knew we'd get answers to all your celeb questions.

Q: How is it that celebrities always have such healthy shiny hair? Do they own some product that we don't?

A: No, they don't. Just because someone has shiny hair doesn't mean it's healthy. There are lots of ways to fake it. "Especially for photo shoots we use a lot of serums and shine sprays in the hair," says Tesinsky. These are products that are either serums (liquidy gels) or sprays that contain ingredients that have a little sparkle to them, so when applied to the hair it looks sparkly too. Another trick that celebs use to make their hair look super-glossy is to blow it straight. "Straight hair always looks shinier than curly hair because it reflects more light," adds Tesinsky.

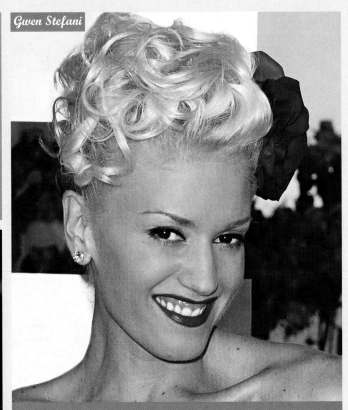

Gwen Stefani

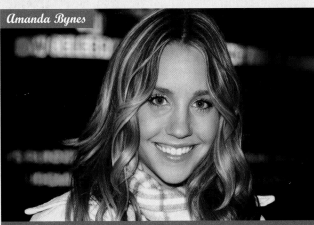

Amanda Bynes

Q. Celebs must blow-dry their hair all the time. How do they stop it from getting all fried and frizzy looking?

A. "Heat styling is the most damaging thing you can do to your hair if it's done wrong," says Weifer. The first trick is to let the hair air-dry a little bit by itself. "If you can start blow-drying your hair when it's barely damp, instead of soaking wet, it's a lot better," she suggests. Also, if you are blowing your hair dry and using a straightening iron, make sure to use a heat-protecting product beforehand—leave-in conditioner is a good one. Finally, when drying, it's important to keep the blow-dryer moving. Never point it at one piece of hair and blast it—this is when hair burns and ends up looking frizzy.

Q. How can someone like Gwen Stefani keep bleaching and bleaching her hair without it falling out of her head?

A. This is where being famous has some serious payoffs. "She probably has a close relationship with a stylist who really knows how to take care of her hair," says Slicker. Bleached hair needs constant conditioning, like using heavy protein deep-conditioning treatments (your hair loses protein when you color it—that's what makes it weak). Also, when you have bleached hair, you need to take precautions, like always wearing a sunscreen on your strands. To protect your own hair from harmful rays, try one of the hair oils on the market that also contain an SPF. Or, in a pinch, you can also use regular body sunscreen on your hair. Just apply it and comb it through so that it's evenly distributed. Hair may look a bit greasy, but that's way better than having it look fried.

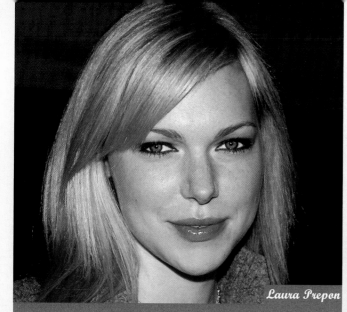

Laura Prepon

Q. What styling product does every star use?

A. "At some point or another, every starlet needs a pomade or wax," says Tesinsky. "It can tame flyaways, add texture to the ends of hair by making it look piece-y, or be used to slick down strands." This stuff feels a little greasy to the touch so when using it only take a pea-sized amount and rub it between your hands, then lightly run hands over hair. To add texture to ends, scrunch up sections of hair in your hands. You can also twist sections around your index finger and let them uncoil (this makes nice messy waves). To tame flyaways or make hair look slick, lightly comb hair after applying.

Q. How do stars get the perfect amount of volume in their hair? Also, once they have all that oomph in their strands, how do they get it to stay?

A. Adding height to your hair isn't as hard as you think. "The trick to getting volume in your hair is to use volumizing products," says Weifer. "Also, keep all the products at the roots of your hair and not on the ends, since that will just weigh your hair down." To start, make sure that hair is about 80 percent dry (damp) because it's much quicker than starting with wet hair. Grab a volumizing spray (these are the easiest to use), and pick up medium chunks of hair (a 2-inch square) and hold it straight up. Spritz hair right at the root. Do this until all of your roots have been sprayed. Next, flip head upside down and blow-dry, using a brush to keep hair smooth as you go. When you're done, flip hair up and avoid brushing it again; just use your fingers to get it how you want it. Tesinsky shares this great tip. "If I'm working on a photo shoot, I'll always put up the girl's hair in a high ponytail on the top of her head. It stays like that while I do her makeup and I'll only take it out right before the photographer is ready. It makes hair look full for a few hours without using any product."

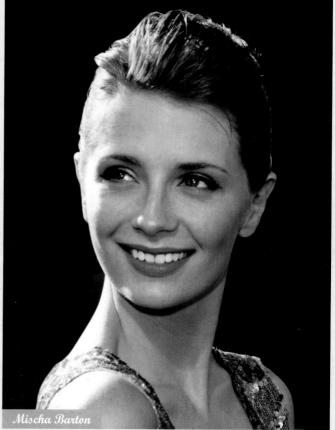

Mischa Barton

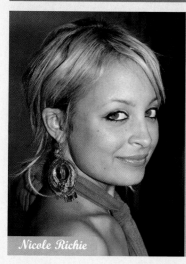

Nicole Richie

Q. Can I still have the same cool hair color as my favorite celeb if I dye my hair at home?

A. All stylists recommend going to a professional the first time you want to dye your hair. "It can be really tricky to know what your hair is going to look like when dyeing it yourself, " says Slicker. "Even if you think your hair is just brown, it always has some hidden undertones to it that might be red or golden, so you need a professional who can figure out what color to use." For example, if you want your hair to look like Drew Barrymore's, your best bet is to bring in lots of pictures to your stylist and have a little show-and-tell. "Sometimes it's hard to know whether a color will look good on you," says Weifer. "Also, if you have dark brown hair and want blond hair like Drew, that means you have to bleach it and then color it. That's a lot of stress on your hair, so maybe we can come up with something different that you'll still love." However, if you are just looking for a temporary change, such as a semi-permanent color that will wash out after 10 shampoos, it's fine to try it at home. Just pick a box where the woman on the front has a color that is fairly close to yours, since these rinses can't do anything too drastic. For more info on what hair dye is right for you, go to "Color-Coded" on page 110.

25 HAIR SECRETS EVERY STAR KNOWS

*W*hether they're strutting down the red carpet or caught by the paparazzi in the middle of the supermarket, celebs always seem to have great hair. Well, that's because every time they show up at a movie premiere or pose for a magazine cover, they have Hollywood's top stylists tending to their strands. With all that primping (not to mention the boatloads of new products they're given), it's no wonder celebs are pretty savvy at fixing their own hair during their downtime. It certainly explains how Kirsten Dunst looks fabulous when she's just walking the dog, or how Drew Barrymore looks awesome leaving a concert. In an attempt to get the lowdown on their insider strand secrets, we grilled Tinseltown's hair experts. Here are some of their favorite hair tips.

1. PART YOUR HAIR SLIGHTLY OFF-CENTER. Have you noticed how celebs love to wear their hair parted in the middle? Hollywood stylist Cheryl Marks, who has worked with **Christina Ricci**, says that there's a sneaky trick to make middle-parted hair look better. When pulling the comb forward from the crown (the top back section of the head), always drag the comb a little to the side so that the part finishes a little bit off-center at your forehead. Your part should always end up a quarter- to half-inch away from the middle of your face. It is more flattering to all face shapes.

2. TAME FRIZZ FREAK-OUTS. If your hair is frizzing out and you haven't got any product, Brian Magallones (who has worked on **Jamie-Lynn Sigler**) says a touch of hand lotion can help. The oils in the lotion will fight frizz by weighing the hair down a bit and getting rid of flyaways. The trick is to use a very small amount (think pea-sized), rub it between your hands, and then smooth it over the top layer of your hair.

3. MAKE STRANDS SPARKLE. If you want your 'do to have a hint of glimmer on a big night out, follow this trick. Take a little bit of loose shimmering powder (either a bronzing powder for your face for dark hair, nude body powder with shimmer for fair hair) and mix it with gel in your hand. Apply the gel to damp hair and style as usual.

4. LESS IS DEFINITELY MORE. Most styling snafus are caused by using too much product. When using gel, use about a quarter-sized amount; for mousse, a tennis ball–sized puff; for serums and waxes, a pea-sized dollop. To make sure that you never suffer from product overload, always start applying products from the back of your head and work your way forward, so you don't end up with too much goo right at the front, where everyone will notice.

5. FIX PRODUCT OVERLOAD BY SPRITZING WITH H$_2$O. If you put too much product in your hair and don't have time to wash it, Ruby Weifer (who's worked on **Mischa Barton**) suggests spritzing it with a little bit of water, brushing it, and giving it a quick blow-dry. This works really well when you've put in too much gel or mousse because the water dilutes the product a little, so your hair won't look as stiff.

6. BLOWDRYING BASICS. Don't start blow-drying your hair when it is soaking wet, says Magallones, wait until hair is 80 percent dry to avoid too much heat styling damage.

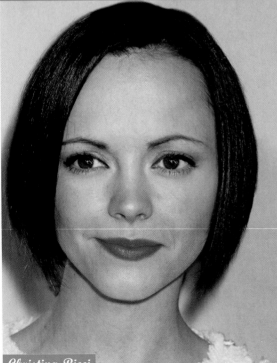
Christina Ricci

7. SEAL IT WITH A CUBE.
What's the quickest shine trick ever? Beverly Hills hair guru Tina Cassaday, who regularly conditions **Liv Tyler's** locks, says that all you need is an ice cube. When you're done styling, take an ice cube out of the freezer and rub it up and down the top layer of your hair. Cassaday says that if you do it while the cube is fresh out of the freezer, the ice won't melt over your hair. The reason this works is that the chill from the cube helps to seal up the hair cuticle (i.e., make it lie flat), which makes hair look super-glossy.

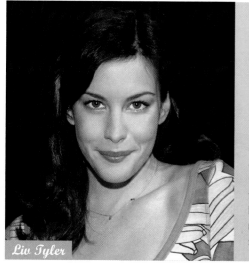
Liv Tyler

8. USE TWO DIFFERENT SIZE CURLING IRONS. Do you love the messy curls of stars like **Sarah Jessica Parker**? The trick is to use two different curling irons—a large-barreled one and a small-barreled one—because naturally curly hair always has different size curls in it. For example, take the larger-barreled curling iron and twist up a couple of sections on the top of your head. Then use the smaller curling iron on the sections around your face. This way your 'do will look glam instead of Goldilocks.

9. GET RID OF THE GREASIES. If your hair sometimes feels a little greasy at the end of the day andyou don't have time for a shower, try this: First, comb your hair with a wide-toothed comb to distribute oil down the hair shaft so it's not as obvious. Next, flip your head upside down and massage your scalp with your fingers to add some volume. Last, spritz on some hairspray because the alcohol in it can absorb some of the scalp oils.

10. SNAG A BEACH LOOK IN A BOTTLE. Lately lots of stars are sporting that back-from-the-beach hair—a little wavy and just unbrushed enough to look cool (**Drew Barrymore** does this look to perfection). Even if you don't live near the ocean, you can sport this look by mixing up a 24-ounce bottle of water with two tablespoons of sea salt in a spray bottle. Spritz hair when it's wet and skip the brushing for this star effect.

11. WAX ON. When using a heavy product like a styling wax, always start applying it at the base of your neck (right where you hair ends in the back) and working your way up and forward. Most people put product on in the front first, and if you apply too much, your 'do is instantly ruined. If you go from the back and work forward, no one will notice.

12. GET MOVIE-SET SLEEK. When stylists need hair to look super smooth on a movie set they use this trick: Squirt a small amount of styling cream in your palm and mix it up using a toothbrush. The heat of your hand heats up the cream. Next, wipe the toothbrush until there's only a tiny amount of product on it and then lightly brush it over the top layer of your hair. This smooths down all those short hairs that tend to sprout out (like around your hairline). This is especially good to do if your hair is pulled back tight and you want it to look sleek.

13. SOFTEN UP AN UPDO. If you love pulling your hair back in a low bun or ponytail, funk it up a bit with a trick that **Jessica Simpson** and **Gwyneth Paltrow** like to wear. When creating your updo, place the bun or ponytail a little left-of-center of the nape of your neck (the lower part in the middle). Also, make a bun a little messy by pulling out a few ends. This way you can see parts of the bun sprouting out from the back when you look at yourself in the mirror. Not only does this look a little cute and different, but it's less severe than just having all of your hair pulled tightly off your face.

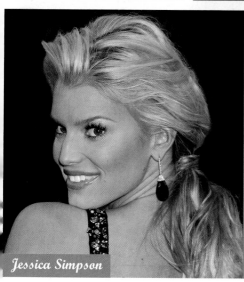
Jessica Simpson

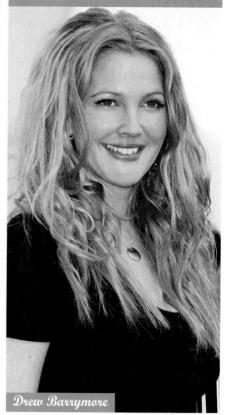
Drew Barrymore

14. LONG LOCK VOLUME TRICK. If your strands are past your shoulders, they can often look flat. Colleen Conway (who has styled **Mandy Moore**) says the best place to add just a touch of volume is at the crown of the head (the highest point in the back). Here's how: Take a one-inch-square section of hair from the crown and hold it straight up. Spritz along the length of the hair with aerosol hairspray (it dries more quickly than a pump version) and roll up into a large Velcro roller. Roll up three more sections the same way, then give them a quick blast with the blow dryer. Remove the rollers, flip hair over, and muss it up with your fingers. Flip hair back right side up and your hair will still be straight, but there will be a flattering lift at the top. This is a great trick if you don't have time to totally redo your style because it only takes about five minutes.

15. MAINTAIN A DYE JOB. How do stars maintain their hair color without the shade turning dull or brassy? Celebs' colorists will often mix up a combo of shampoo and a little bit of the hair color for the celeb to take home. Every couple of weeks she can lather up with the stuff and give her color a little kick. Ask your colorist about doing the same if you're interested in changing your hair hue.

16. DARK TRESS SECRET. Stars like **Christina Aguilera**, who have light hair but occasionally like to color it darker, can have trouble camouflaging their blond roots. Carla Gentile, owner of Steam Salon (where **Lauren Ambrose** has been spotted), says that in a pinch you can use a dab of black mascara to hide light roots and help them to blend with your darker locks. Apply a dab using the wand, and then comb it out so the mascara won't look clumpy.

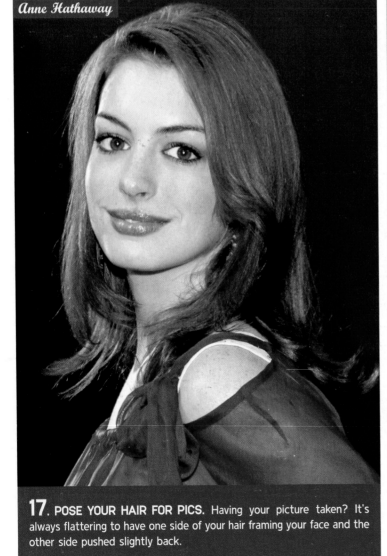

Anne Hathaway

18. FRAME YOUR FACE. When cutting bangs, it's more flattering for all face shapes to have them sloping down a bit at the sides than to just be cut straight across.

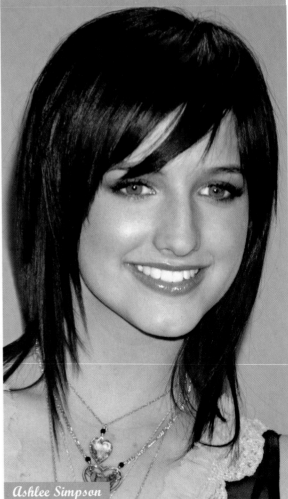

Ashlee Simpson

17. POSE YOUR HAIR FOR PICS. Having your picture taken? It's always flattering to have one side of your hair framing your face and the other side pushed slightly back.

19. STOP SNAGGING ELASTIC BANDS. To stop elastic bands from getting tangled up in your hair and breaking your strands, cover them in a small amount of conditioner and they'll slip on and off easily.

20. GROWING OUT THE EASY WAY. Yes, it's torture growing out a short 'do, but there are ways to make it less painful. Keep the ends cut fairly blunt—that means getting regular trims (Kimberly Kimble does this with **Beyoncé** to keep her ends sharp and fresh-looking). The longer hair goes without a tiny chop, the more uneven and frayed looking the tips get, which gives the illusion of it being shorter and less thick. "Also, not cutting your hair doesn't make it grow any faster," says Kimble.

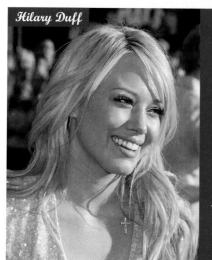

Hilary Duff

21. LONGER HAIR IS JUST A SHOPPING TRIP AWAY. How is it that famous hairdos seem to grow so much quicker than ours? Well, the reason is often hair extensions (**Hilary Duff** and **Paris Hilton** have been seen sporting them). While stars use stylists to weave their fake hair in, you can easily go to the drugstore and buy some fake pieces that can just be clipped onto your hair or attached like a ponytail. Perfect for a fun night out!

22. LIGHTEN UP ON THE HAIRSPRAY. If you need to give your hair a quick spritz during the day, don't just keep piling on more hairspray—after a few applications, your 'do will start to look a little crispy. Instead, grab a round or paddle brush, spritz the spray onto the bristles, and use that to add product to your tresses by gently brushing hair into place.

23. AVOID FRIZZIES AND KNOTS. Don't rub your head with a towel—it musses up your strands. Instead, grab a section of your hair in a towel and just squeeze out the moisture with your hands. This also cuts your combing time in half.

24. HIDE SMELLY HAIR ODORS. Hair is really susceptible to absorbing all sorts of odors, so if you've been out with your friends for some burgers and fries, don't be surprised if your strands smell "supersized." While there are hair fragrances on the market, you can also mask the odor by spritzing your regular fragrance up in the air right in front of your body, and then walking through the mist. Enough of the scent will fall on your strands to help hide the odor.

25. DON'T BE AFRAID TO EXPERIMENT. Especially if you don't want to cut your hair, it's easy to create tons of different styles. Just look at **Jennifer Lopez**—one minute it's in long sexy waves, the next in a sleek ponytail or a sweetly girlish 'do. Learn to experiment with your blow-dryer and different products. Just like your makeup, hair makes a huge statement about your personality, so don't be afraid to let it show the world how you really feel.

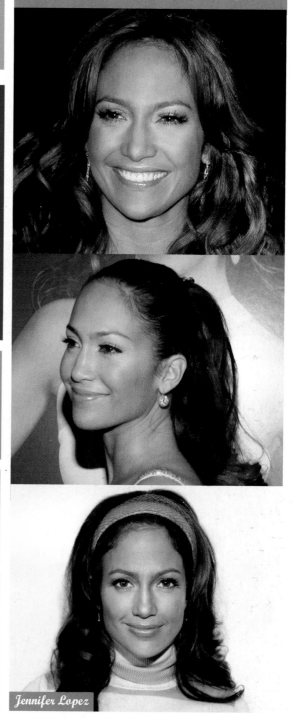

Jennifer Lopez

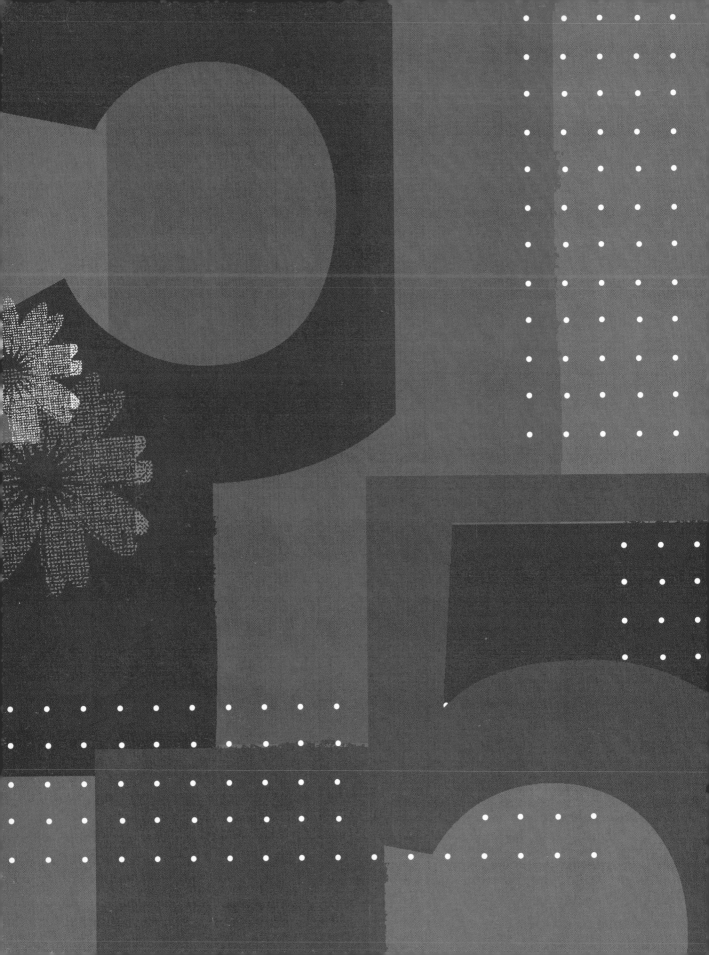

chapter five

FAB FINISHING TOUCHES

all the details you need to steal the spotlight

GLAM BODY BASICS

*W*hoever said "it's all in the details" was right. Paying attention to small things like hair removal, self-tanner application, and sun protection plays a big role in looking your best. You walk a little taller when every inch of you is perfectly groomed.

THE BEST WAYS TO BANISH UNWANTED FUZZ

SHAVING

WHAT IT IS: A razor cuts hair off at your skin's surface.

HOW OFTEN YOU HAVE TO DO IT: Hair grows back in one to four days.

WHAT IT'S GOOD FOR: It's a quick and easy way to remove hair on your legs or underarms. (NEVER EVER shave your face or you will look even hairier when the fuzz grows back.)

WATCH OUT: The straight edge of a razor can be dangerous in awkward areas, like your bikini zone. Shaving can also make hair grow back coarser because the razor chops hair off at the center of the shaft, where hair is thick.

TIP: Always shave in the shower, when skin and hair are soft from the heat. Use a fresh razor blade with tons of shaving cream or gel for a super-smooth surface. COST: $

DEPILATORY LOTIONS

WHAT IT IS: Chemicals dissolve hair at your skin's surface.

HOW OFTEN YOU HAVE TO DO IT: Hair grows back in three to seven days.

WHAT IT'S GOOD FOR: Lotions are better for hard-to-reach areas and those with uneven surfaces that a razor can easily nick, like your bikini zone. Hair grows back less coarsely than with a razor, so lotions are also good for areas like your upper lip or your chin.

WATCH OUT: If you don't wash lotions off within the recommended time, they can be irritating. (If you don't get all the fuzz off in your first try, wait at least a day before trying again, or you can really irritate your skin.)

TIP: Follow up hair removal with a medicated gel or lotion to soothe itching, bumps, and redness. COST: $

COOL AND WARM WAXES

WHAT IT IS: Waxes pull hair out from the follicles.

HOW OFTEN YOU HAVE TO DO IT: You will be bare of hair for up to six weeks.

WHAT IT'S GOOD FOR: Safe to use on your upper lip, between your eyebrows, and on your underarms, bikini area, and legs. Waxes leave you looking totally hairless, with no dark spots for a long time.

WATCH OUT: They can be irritating, especially if you have sensitive skin. Waxing can also lead to ingrown hairs.

TIP: When waxing, pull your skin taut and pull the strip or cloth in the opposite direction of hair growth. COST: $$

LASERS

WHAT IT IS: A laser destroys hair follicles so hair stops growing.

HOW OFTEN YOU HAVE TO DO IT: Hair might come back in three to five years but results can last forever for a lucky few.

WHAT IT'S GOOD FOR: You might never have to think about hair removal again on your upper lip, underarms, legs, and bikini zone.

WATCH OUT: It's super-pricy and the lasers can make your skin look permanently blotchy.

TIP: Don't wax or tweeze first; you need to have full hair growth for it to be effective. Also, stick to MDs; laser procedures are often available from aestheticians, but they are not as well trained as a dermatologist or doctor—and you can get burned if the procedure is done incorrectly. COST: $$$$

ELECTROLYSIS

WHAT IT IS: An electrical needle destroys your hair follicles to stop hair growth.

HOW OFTEN YOU HAVE TO DO IT: Once—it's permanent.

WHAT IT'S GOOD FOR: The process is very precise, so you can remove any hair, anywhere.

WATCH OUT: If done incorrectly, it can be painful and can lead to scarring.

TIP: This procedure should be done by a licensed dermatologist or a medical doctor trained in the procedure. COST: $$$

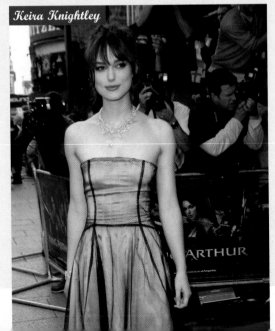

Keira Knightley

THE BEST WAY TO FAKE A TAN

YOUR SELF-TANNER OPTIONS:

• **LOTIONS:** Rich in moisturizers, self-tanning lotions soften skin as they tan. They can be thick, so be sure to rub them in completely and allow them to dry for up to an hour to make sure the tanner is evenly distributed.

• **SPRAYS:** Sprays are the quickest way to go bronze and they are virtually goof-proof. But don't just spritz and go—sprays still need to be rubbed in.

• **TINTED GELS:** Tinted gels make even color instant and easy—you'll be sun-kissed on the spot. Plus, even distribution of color is a snap because you can see exactly where you've applied color and where you haven't. Tip: Use tinted bronzing gels to cover up tan lines and strap marks.

• **FOAMS:** Foams are light, just like whipped cream, and easy to apply evenly over your skin. They also dry fairly fast.

Tip: Self-tanning is best when done with your friends, since you can't reach every part of your body by yourself—like the center of your back. So before getting started, make a few calls, and invite the girls over for an afternoon of fake-baking.

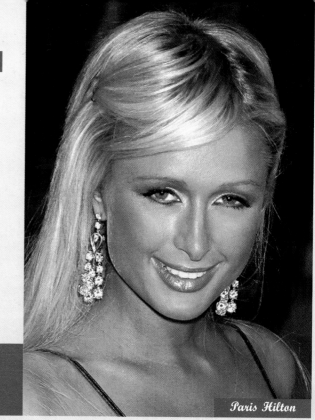

Paris Hilton

1. Exfoliate your entire body—especially your knees and elbows, where skin is rougher—so skin is silky soft and self-tanner will go on splotch-free.

2. Dry your skin completely and slip your hands into thin disposable latex gloves (available at any drugstore) so you won't stain your fingers and nails—a surefire giveaway that you're a phony.

3. Start by applying self-tanner to your legs and down onto the tops of your feet. Pat dry your knees and ankles with a tissue to prevent splotches.

4. Next, do your arms, following the same routine. Tissue-dry elbows. Leave hands tanner-free for now.

5. Coat your chest and tummy (don't forget your sides), then your face and ears.

6. Get a pal to rub tanner over your back.

7. For hands, remove one glove and use your gloved hand to apply tanner to the top of your hand and fingers. Remove tanner from your knuckles with a tissue. Wait 15 minutes or until your tanned hand is dry to the touch; replace the rubber glove. Remove the other glove and repeat on other hand.

8. Don't sit down until your body is completely dry—anywhere from almost immediately to 15 minutes. You be the judge (some self tanners take longer to dry).

9. Reapply as necessary to stay bronzed and beautiful.

THE BEST WAY TO GET SAFE SUN

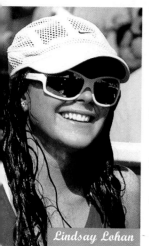

Lindsay Lohan

1. When hitting the beach or pool, always coat your entire body with a generous amount of broad spectrum, water-resistant sunscreen with at least SPF 15; look for zinc oxide or Parsol® 1789 in the ingredients.

2. Protect your face with oil-free SPF 15-and-higher sunscreens; don't forget your ears, nose, the part in your hairline, and lips.

3. Show off sun-savvy chic with a wide-brimmed hat and sunglasses with UV protection.

4. If you know you'll be sweating, coat yourself with a sweat-proof sunblock.

5. Always apply sunscreen 30 minutes before you go outside, giving it time to be absorbed into your skin; reapply sunscreen every two hours and after swimming.

6. Every day, rain or shine, slather on body and face moisturizers that contain SPF 15. Damaging sun rays can shoot through your clothing and harm your skin—a white T-shirt only has an SPF of 8.

7. Be extra careful in the sun if you have pale skin, freckles, light eyes, blond or red hair, or are on antibiotics.

10 WAYS TO GET RED-CARPET CONFIDENCE

Stars strut down the red carpet looking like they are on top of the world: cool, calm and collected all the time. You know what we mean–they're always smiling, back perfectly straight, and never a misstep (without ever looking at the ground!). And they pull it all off while millions of fans check them out and cameras flash in their faces.

These beauty tips are of a different kind–they have to do with what you're feeling inside and how those feelings are reflected on the outside. They'll help you be that girl who has a confident strut with great posture, who looks you in the eye when she speaks, and lights up a room when she smiles because she is broadcasting confidence. You'll be even more spectacular than you already are–because confidence equals beauty. Here's how to show the world just how great you are!

You can tell these celebs are oozing confidence. Here's why:

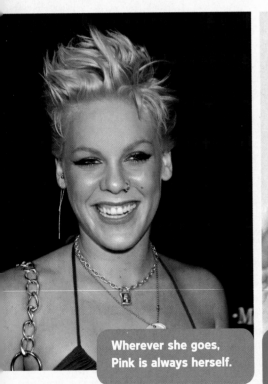

Wherever she goes, Pink is always herself.

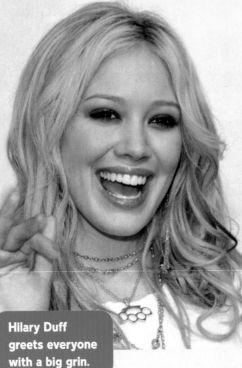

Hilary Duff greets everyone with a big grin.

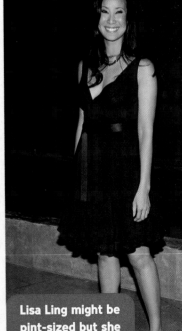

Lisa Ling might be pint-sized but she stands tall with a straight back.

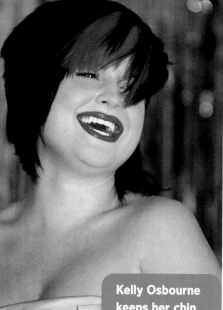

We would all love to have Jennifer's tresses, but she doesn't let them take over her life—or her face.

Kelly Osbourne keeps her chin up, even on rainy days.

Act Like a Star! Here's How:

1. SMILE! Nothing makes you look more self-assured—and beautiful!—than a big, bright, beaming smile.

2. MAKE EYE CONTACT. When you look the person that you are speaking to or listening to in the eye, you are telling them that you care about them, that they are important to you, and that you are cool enough, and self-assured enough, to let them know it.

3. STAND UP STRAIGHT. Face the world standing tall and you broadcast that you're happy and secure. Stretch up to your full height—imagine a string is pulling the center of the top of your head up to the sky. (Slouchers look passive, insecure, and radiate "don't look at me" vibes.)

4. HOLD YOUR CHIN UP HIGH. Holding your chin so it juts straight ahead is the perfect way to say "I am totally confident." When chatting, you'll seem enthralled. And, in class, holding your chin up will make you look like you're paying attention, even if you're not!

5. DON'T HIDE BEHIND YOUR HAIR. Pull your hair back into a pony or shove it behind your ears so you can face the day—and your friends, family, and teachers—head-on.

6. KEEP NERVOUS HABITS UNDER CONTROL. The easiest way to look cool and calm is to avoid public displays of stressed-out behavior like nail biting, cuticle picking, zit picking, or tress twisting.

7. DON'T FIDGET. Ever catch yourself shaking your leg or tapping your foot like mad in class? You really need to try to stop immediately, even if you are bored out of your mind. Easier said than done? Try meditation or amp up your regular exercise routine.

8. DON'T GO OUT IN PUBLIC LOOKING LIKE A SLOB. No matter your look, whether it's preppy chic, boho mellow, or even all-out grunge, take the time to put yourself together so your personal style shows through.

9. BE GENEROUS WITH COMPLIMENTS—WHEN THEY ARE TRUE. Nothing takes more confidence than giving someone a compliment. Saying "Your haircut looks so cute!" or "I love that shirt!" makes your pal feel good and shows you feel good about yourself.

10. TELL THE TRUTH. Hey—you are so interesting and cool that you can interest people simply by telling the truth. The key is to live a life you're psyched to tell the world about. You'll have every reason to be confident—and it will shine through!!

SAY CHEESE!

Stars like Jessica Simpson, Hilary Duff, and Beyoncé are always flashing pearly white, camera-worthy grins. That's because they know a secret. There's nothing more powerful than a smile. When someone flashes one your way, it just makes you feel great.

And there's something else that's powerful about a smile. Give the world your biggest and brightest grin, and it will not only make you look happy on the outside, it is guaranteed to make you feel happy inside too. Why not give it a try on the next gloomy day that comes your way? Force a grin and your day might just become a wee bit brighter! Smiling is a surefire way to make yourself look and feel beautiful–in an instant. Read on to learn about all the inexpensive and easy ways you can make your smile shine like the stars'!

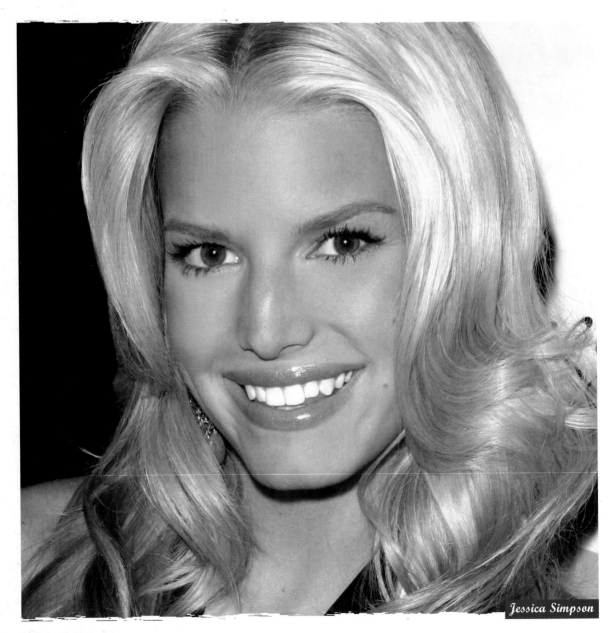

Jessica Simpson

BRIGHTEN YOUR SMILE!

For full-on, easy, at-home whitening you've got three choices:

1. USE A WHITENING TOOTHPASTE AND LEARN TO BRUSH THE RIGHT WAY.

Polish your teeth and brush away stains twice a day with a whitening toothpaste that's packed with peroxide. These days most dentists are giving electric brushes two thumbs up. They get teeth squeaky clean, plus they massage and clear out the gum line. Whether you like to use an electric or manual toothbrush, learn to hold it correctly. "Hold the brush at a 45-degree angle to your gums, and brush in a circular motion, so your gums get some TLC too," advises Jennifer Salzer, DDS, a NYC dentist who works on tons of celebs. She adds, "keep brushing away for at least two minutes—about as long as a song lasts on the radio—to let the paste really go to work." Pressing down hard with the toothbrush won't get your teeth whiter; in fact, it can hurt you in the long run by damaging gums and wearing away enamel, so use a light hand.

If you're wearing braces, you need to pay special attention to your teeth. "Braces act like magnets for food and plaque, both of which can stain," says Salzer. Brush after every meal, and follow up with mouthwash, which can help dislodge some of the leftovers from between your tracks.

2. TURN UP YOUR WHITENESS WATTAGE WITH WHITENING STRIPS.

Whitening strips containing peroxide stick snugly to your teeth and stay on your teeth for about 30 minutes (much longer than a whitening toothpaste), so they'll make your teeth whiter by a few shades. Follow the directions on the package when you put them on, and be sure to push them into the creases between your teeth for even coverage. "Steer clear of your gums, however, because the peroxide can irritate them, making them red and puffy," explains Steven Fox, DDS, a cosmetic dentist in New York City. Warning: Don't be tempted to leave the strips on for longer than the amount of time that is recommended on the package. Whitening can make your teeth very sensitive (especially to extreme temperatures).

3. SLICK ON WHITENING GELS FOR A BRIGHT WHITE.

Brush-on whitening gels also contain peroxide to whiten teeth a few shades. "While these brush-on gels seem easier to apply than a strip, they can still be tricky," warns Fox. Carefully brush the gel over one tooth at a time, and avoid the gum line at all costs (again, peroxide can be irritating). Keep your mouth open and still for about 30 seconds after application to give the gel time to dry and set in place. Otherwise, the gel can easily be washed away with saliva and even irritate your throat.

→ QUIZ: WHAT'S SO FUNNY?

EACH ONE OF THESE PEARLY WHITE GRINS BELONGS TO A CELEBRITY. MATCH THE SMILE WITH THE STAR.

1. LINDSAY LOHAN
2. BRITNEY SPEARS
3. ANNE HATHAWAY
4. JESSICA BIEL
5. KATE HUDSON

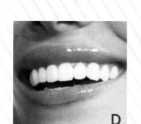
A

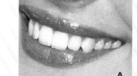
B

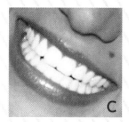
C

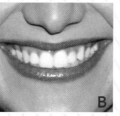
D

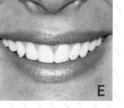
E

ANSWER KEY: 1E; 2C; 3A; 4D; 5B

FAMOUS NAILS

*T*here's nothing like a manicure or pedicure to lift a girl's spirits or change the way she looks at the world. Where would Reese Witherspoon's character in **Legally Blonde** have been without her best friend/manicurist? There are definitely girls out there who will swear they think better when their digits are looking their best. Certainly you have to consider the terrific first impression you make with a great pair of clean, well-manicured hands—and that's even before you've opened your mouth! These days, there's a look and color for every mood from classic pale pinks, nudes, or reds to wilder "anything goes" colors like green, blue, or yellow.

Elsbeth Schuetz, who does the nails of stars such as Jessica Simpson, Paris Hilton, Kirsten Dunst, and Courtney Cox Arquette, gives you the 411 on DIY manis and pedis, plus the scoop on how the celebs are painting their nails.

STAR STYLE

ONCE YOU HAVE THE BASICS DOWN, LET SCHUETZ GIVE YOU THE INSIDE SCOOP ON SOME OF THE COOL WAYS SHE'S DECORATED A FEW OF HER STAR CLIENTS' NAILS.

Paris Hilton

Schuetz has dressed up Paris' fingernails in hearts with silver linings. Here's how to do it.

What You'll Need
- ❑ WHITE OR CANDY PINK NAIL POLISH
- ❑ RED NAIL POLISH
- ❑ TINY PAINTBRUSH, (FROM A CRAFT OR ART-SUPPLY STORE)
- ❑ TOOTHPICK
- ❑ LARGE-SIZED SILVER GLITTER

How to Do It

1. Paint your nails in either white or candy pink nail polish; let dry.

2. Dip the tiny brush into red nail polish (if the bristles won't fit in the bottle, pour some polish onto tin foil and lift it from there with the brush; just be sure there is only the tiniest bit of polish on the brush—painting itsy-bitsy hearts is a precise business!). Take a few practice twirls on paper before trying it on your nails.

3. On your thumbnail (the largest surface area and therefore the easiest to work on) paint a little heart.

4. While the heart is still wet, lick the tip of a toothpick to make it sticky (uncooked spaghetti works great too, 'cause it gets extra, extra sticky), pick up one sparkly speck, and place it on the outline of your heart. Keep at it until the heart is totally lined.

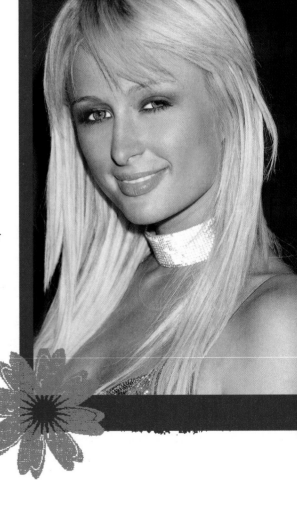

DO-IT-YOURSELF PEDICURES

What You'll Need
- ❏ NAIL POLISH REMOVER
- ❏ TOENAIL CLIPPERS
- ❏ EMERY BOARD
- ❏ PUMICE STONE
- ❏ FOOT SCRUB
- ❏ FOOT CREAM
- ❏ ASTRINGENT
- ❏ RUBBER TOE SEPARATOR OR TISSUE PAPER
- ❏ BASE COAT
- ❏ NAIL POLISH IN THE COLOR OF YOUR CHOICE
- ❏ CLEAR NAIL POLISH

How to Do It
1. Clear your nails of any polish with nail polish remover. Use toenail clippers (which are larger than fingernail clippers) to cut toenails straight across; round the sides very slightly with an emery board (otherwise you can cause ingrown toenails). Don't file in a sawing motion; instead, "file repeatedly in one direction," says Schuetz.

DO-IT-YOURSELF MANICURES

What You'll Need
- ❏ NAIL POLISH REMOVER
- ❏ GENTLE SOAP
- ❏ TABLE SALT
- ❏ CUTICLE OR OLIVE OIL
- ❏ RUBBER-TIPPED ORANGE STICK
- ❏ EMERY BOARD
- ❏ BASE COAT
- ❏ NAIL POLISH IN THE COLOR OF YOUR CHOICE
- ❏ CLEAR NAIL POLISH

How to Do It
1. Make a clean start. "Clear your nails of any old polish or residue with nail polish remover," says Schuetz. "Then wash your hands with gentle soap and water. "

2. Soften your cuticle (the thin line of skin at the base of your nails). Soak fingers in a bowl of salty, warm water—you can use a dash of table salt—for three to five minutes.

3. Rub cuticle oil—olive oil will do the trick too—into your nail beds (the area where your nails grow from your fingers) and gently push back your cuticles with a rubber-tipped orange stick. Don't cut your cuticles; they help protect nails. And, even worse, the more you cut cuticles, the more rough and raggedy they grow back.

2. Buff any rough, dead skin or calluses on dry feet with a pumice stone. Take a pumice stone (which typically is a loose gray stone or is attached to a handle) and gently rub it back and forth over rough patches for a few minutes. Next, soak feet in warm, sudsy water and rub off the rest of the dead skin with a foot scrub containing exfoliants like sphere beads or nuts. (Nuts, which aren't always good for your face because they can be irritating, are okay to use on your feet, since the skin is thicker and stronger.) Give tootsies a good rub and rinse clean.

3. Dry your feet and coat them—toe to sole—with a foot cream. Next, wipe each toenail clean with an astringent-soaked tissue so your nails aren't covered with a slippery film of cream.

4. Separate toes with a toe separator (it looks like a rubber comb) or take a twisted length of facial tissue and weave it though toes to prevent nail polish smudges. Apply a clear base coat.

5. Next, top it with your fave polish, applying one swipe down the middle followed by a swipe on each side of your nail. Let dry for five minutes, then apply a second coat. To make color last, top off nails with a clear topcoat.

4. Use an emery board to file your tips into an oval or square shape. Always file in one direction; a back and forth sawing motion can rip your nails. Tip: "If you have weak nails that tend to break, go for the square shape, which is stronger," says Schuetz.

5. Apply a base coat to hold polish on longer and keep the color from staining your nails. Brush a single stroke down the center of your nail, then one down each side, avoiding your cuticles and skin. Let dry.

6. Apply a single thin, even coat of colored polish to each finger using the same method you used for the base coat; apply a second coat of colored polish starting with the first finger you polished. Try not to touch the polish to your skin or cuticle—it will make the polish chip faster.

7. "Brush on a clear topcoat to protect polish from chipping and peeling, and to give color a super-shiny finish," says Schuetz.

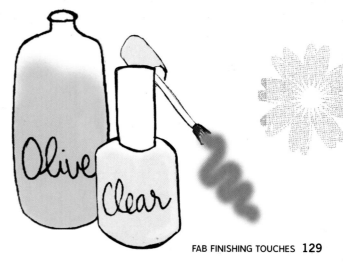

Jessica Simpson

For an Oscar bash, Schuetz monogrammed Jessica's thumbnail with her husband Nick's initials.

What You'll Need
- ☐ PALE PINK AND WHITE NAIL POLISHES
- ☐ TINY PAINTBRUSH
- ☐ TOOTHPICK
- ☐ RHINESTONES

How to Do It

1. Paint your nails with two coats of pale pink polish; let dry.

2. Dip the tiny brush into the white polish, tap off any excess, and swivel the bristles against the top of bottle to create a point. (If the brush doesn't fit in the bottle, pour some polish onto foil and lift it from there with the brush.)

3. On your thumbnail (the largest surface area and therefore the easiest to work on), paint initials. They don't have to be your boyfriend's; they could be your own, your best friend's, or even your pet's.

4. Give the monogram some sparkle by adding a rhinestone. Before the polish dries, lick the end of a toothpick so it's sticky and use it to pick up a rhinestone. Place the sparkler on one of the letters.

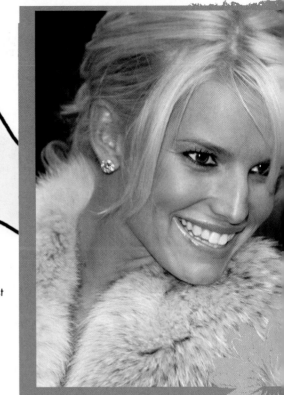

Kirsten Dunst

Want to keep your finger on the pulse of current events? It's easy with newsprint nails, a favorite look of Kirsten Dunst's.

What You'll Need
- ☐ WHITE OPAQUE NAIL POLISH
- ☐ NEWSPAPER
- ☐ SCISSORS
- ☐ SPRAY NAIL CLEANSER THAT CONTAINS ACETONE
- ☐ CLEAR TOPCOAT POLISH

How to Do It

1. Paint your nails with two coats of opaque white polish; let dry completely.

2. Flip though the newspaper and find type you like. Cut it out. Choose letters or symbols that will still make sense flipped, since the impression on your nail will come out in reverse. For example, "XOXO" is foolproof.

3. Give the nails that you plan to decorate a clean sweep with spray nail cleanser (it's the same formulation as the kind that comes in bottles or towelettes but is in a spray bottle). Spritz a few shots of spray on your nails.

4. While the nail is damp with spray cleanser, press the newsprint facedown and hold for 10 seconds, so your chosen words come in contact with your nail and the print comes off on the white polish. Carefully lift up the sheet of type.

5. Wait a few minutes for your nails to dry, then apply a clear topcoat to keep everything in place.

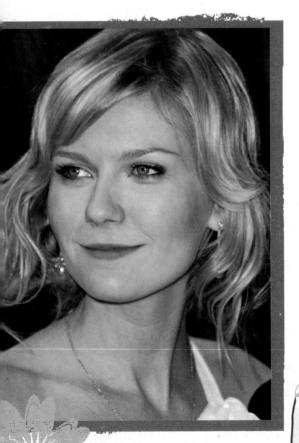

Courteney Cox Arquette

Create far-out textures and patterns on your nails just like the ones worn by Courteney Cox Arquette with the dab of a sponge.

What You'll Need
- ❑ HIGH-SHINE RED, SILVER, AND GOLD NAIL POLISHES
- ❑ FOIL
- ❑ SMALL SQUARE-INCH PIECES CUT FROM A NEW SPONGE (THE KITCHEN VARIETY WILL WORK)
- ❑ TOOTHPICK
- ❑ RHINESTONES

How to Do It

1. Paint your nails with two coats of the red nail polish; let dry.

2. Pour a dime-sized dollop of the gold polish onto a small piece of foil, so it is easier to get at with the sponge.

3. Dip the end of the sponge into it, then dab your nails to create a far-out texture; let dry.

4. Repeat with the silver polish.

5. While the silver polish is still wet, lick a toothpick and pick up a rhinestone, which you can place anywhere while the polish is still drying (and sticky).

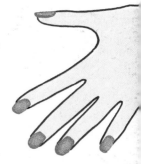

SUPER SIMPLE NAIL CARE TIPS

- To remove polish stains or yellowing, soak nails in warm water saturated with lemon juice.

- To keep nails strong and prevent them from breaking, cut them short, about as long as the top of your finger.

- To make manicures last longer, wear rubber gloves when washing dishes. Dish detergent can make polish fade or change color.

- To avoid air bubbles in your nail polish, don't shake the bottle. Instead, roll it gently in the palms of your hands before applying.

QUIZ: WHAT IS YOUR FRAGRANCE PERSONALITY?

*T*here are so many different kinds of perfumes and fragrances out there: some are flowery, others are fruity or citrusy, and still others are spicy. And since the fragrance you spritz on your wrists says a lot about you, pick the right message in a bottle—or you could end up sending out the wrong signal. In order to help you discover what kind of scents you like, we created this fragrance finder quiz. It will not only help you discover your fragrance personality type, it will match you with the celeb who best personifies your scent match.

1. YOUR FAVORITE TYPE OF COMFORT FOOD IS . . .
A) Light and simple, like pasta
B) Sweet, like angel food cake
C) Spicy, like Chinese takeout
D) Fruity, like apples and oranges

2. YOU ALWAYS GULP DOWN . . .
A) Ice-cold water
B) A chocolate milk shake
C) Herbal tea
D) A fruit smoothie

3. YOU GET YOUR BODY SQUEAKY CLEAN WITH . . .
A) A bar of deodorant soap that smells like evergreen
B) Bubble bath that smells like a garden of flowers
C) A liquid cleanser that is packed with woodsy-smelling scents
D) A pink pouf filled with a fruity fragranced wash

4. WHEN YOU SMELL _____, YOU CAN'T HELP BUT SMILE.
A) Freshly squeezed lemonade
B) A bouquet of roses
C) Incense
D) An apple you just bit into

5. YOUR FAVORITE CLOTHING FABRIC TO WEAR IS . . .
A) Cotton, like sweats and an old T-shirt. Jennifer Aniston Lives in cotton—except when winning awards!
B) Silk, like a silky pink robe—very Reese Witherspoon in *Legally Blonde*.
C) Denim, like in an outfit inspired by Norah Jones—blue jeans and an Indian-print shirt.
D) Cashmere—a pink cashmere sweater can make any outfit look well put together. Kirsten Dunst throws one on with jeans and looks like a million bucks.

6. YOUR FAVORITE COLORS TO WEAR ARE . . .
A) Whites, creams, and neutrals, like Scarlett Johansson
B) Pastels, like pale pink and green, favorites of Natalie Portman
C) Rich jewel tones, like deep red and purple, like Nicole Richie
D) Brights, like kelly green and royal blue—think Gwen Stefani

7. YOUR FAVORITE SEASON IS . . .
A) Summer
B) Spring
C) Fall
D) Winter

8. YOU WEAR PERFUME TO . . .
A) Feel fresh throughout the day
B) Up your feminine appeal—it's fun being girly
C) Leave a lingering memory of yourself wherever you go
D) Show everyone you know the latest "in" scent

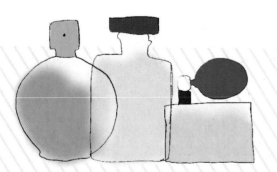

Fragrance Finder Key

IF YOU PICKED MOSTLY As . . .

FRAGRANCE PERSONALITY: YOU ARE A SPORTY GAL, LIKE SERENA WILLIAMS

FRAGRANCE FINDS: Try fresh green and citrus scents, like green leaves, basil, chamomile, grass, and pine. Fragrance-filled body washes and moisture lotions will fit your active lifestyle.

IF YOU PICKED MOSTLY Bs . . .

FRAGRANCE PERSONALITY: YOU ARE A TRUE ROMANTIC, LIKE JESSICA SIMPSON

FRAGRANCE FINDS: Dress up your skin with flowery fragrances that contain ingredients like rose, tuberose, gardenia, jasmine, and hyacinth. To feel lovely, dab a *parfum* formula (the strongest scent option since it is pure fragrance with nothing to water it down) onto your wrists and neck.

IF YOU PICKED MOSTLY Cs . . .

FRAGRANCE PERSONALITY: YOU ARE A BOHEMIAN BABE, LIKE VANESSA CARLTON

FRAGRANCE FINDS: Search out spicy Oriental fragrances that contain amber, musk, vanilla, ginger, sandalwood, and bergamot. Fragrance oils and balms can be massaged into your skin for a total sensory experience.

IF YOU PICKED MOSTLY Ds . . .

FRAGRANCE PERSONALITY: YOU ARE A SUPER-TRENDY GIRL, LIKE CHRISTINA AGUILERA

FRAGRANCE FINDS: Pick modern, fruity fragrances, like lemon, peach, orange, and grape-fruit. Spritz your bod with an eau de toilette spray, which is lighter (and less expensive) than a *parfum* and can be sprayed all over so you smell head-to-toe yummy.

FRAGRANCE NOTES

Before you spritz your scent-sational find, check out these fragrance facts.

✱ To make a fragrance last as long as possible, keep it away from extreme cold (like on a windowsill in the winter) and heat (like in your bathroom when it's steamy from a shower).

✱ To smell great throughout the day, layer your fragrance pick. Try using a body wash, followed by moisturizer, and then the actual fragrance, all in the same scent.

✱ For pretty-smelling clothes, tuck fragrant sachet bags or homemade perfume-soaked cotton bundles tied with ribbon in drawers.

✱ Spray perfume onto your ironing board before pressing your pants and blouses.

✱ Eat spicy, high-fat foods, like Thai or Chinese, to make your fragrance smell more intense.

✱ You know you are wearing too much fragrance if someone farther than an arm's length away from you can smell it.

chapter six

MORE BEAUTY
SCOOP

extra celebrity fun

BEAUTY HOROSCOPES

*W*hat's your astro-tude when it comes to beauty? We looked to the stars (in the sky) and matched them with another kind of star (the Hollywood kind) for a little peek into what type of person you are. As well as getting some insight into your personality, each sign also has its own style vibe. So whether you're a bold Leo or a dreamy Pisces, there's a look out there that's just right for you. Read on for tons of info on what kind of person you are, what's the best thing about you, as well as how to showcase all your special features—whether it's your smiling eyes or energetic attitude. Plus, there are tons of tips on what beauty loot will look fabulous on you.

Aries ♈ MARCH 21–APRIL 20

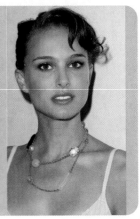

STAR SIBLING: *Reese Witherspoon*

WHO YOU ARE: You guys are the Energizer Bunny of the zodiac! People who know you well would say that you are spontaneous, energetic, and outgoing. If there is an award for school spirit at your school, we're pretty sure that you are in the final running. Plus, your optimistic attitude makes everyone gravitate to you.

YOUR BEAUTY OUTLOOK: When it comes to beauty routines, rams are pretty low-maintenance. You normally spend no more than 10 to 20 minutes getting ready—you tend to like the same look all the time. But since you're comfortable in the limelight, why not take it one step further and make your looks become as one-of-a-kind as your attitude? Try something bold and beautiful like a line of colored eyeliner across your top lash line or a quirky hair accessory in your ponytail.

Taurus ♉ APRIL 21–MAY 21

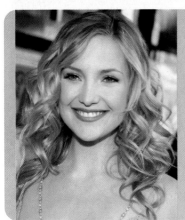

STAR SIBLING: *Kate Hudson*

WHO YOU ARE: You are one of the most loyal and warm signs, so everyone wants to be your friend. Because of this, one of your best features is your killer smile. But at the same time, you don't have the need to be the life of the party, and prefer small gatherings with a couple of close friends. You are also super-patient and have a huge amount of willpower.

YOUR BEAUTY OUTLOOK: Since your grin is your main thing, why not enhance it even more by trying a bright lipstick or gloss? The main rule to remember when wearing a standout pout is keep the rest of your face fairly simple (no bright-colored shadows or sparkly cheeks). When it comes to products, you're into having the latest cool brands, but be choosy when buying. Our advice is to go cheap on basic stuff like mascara so you can splurge on something special, like a new fragrance or some great shampoo and conditioner.

Gemini ♊ MAY 22–JUNE 22

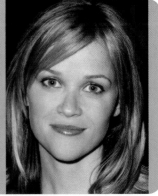

STAR SIBLING: *Natalie Portman*

WHO YOU ARE: If you had to pick between beauty or brains, you'd definitely pick smarts. Geminis are the most quick-witted sign of the zodiac, so people love you for your witty conversations and snappy comebacks. You're are also very easygoing and have no problem adapting to new places or people; actually, you are quite happy the more your routine changes, since Geminis can get bored easily.

YOUR BEAUTY OUTLOOK: Twins like to change their looks quite a lot. While we applaud your creative spirit, be careful. For example, if you want to keep switching up your hair color, use a semi-permanent shade that only lasts for a few weeks (you'll be ready for a change by then) since these won't damage your hair. If you want a drastic change, consult a professional colorist. Another great way to switch up your style is to become your own mix master—stock up on a lip gloss palette that has a few different shades in it, so you can swirl a few together and create your own new hue.

Cancer ♋ JUNE 23–JULY 23

STAR SIBLING: *Lindsay Lohan*

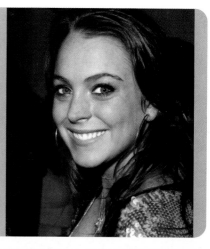

WHO YOU ARE: You are a true earth mother, and the most caring and nurturing sign of the zodiac. You might come across as quiet and reserved sometimes, but that's only because there is so much going on in your head, thanks to that wonderful imagination. Your emotions can also change with the wind—one minute you're frustrated by homework, and the next you turn into a total mushy mess if your crush walks by. You are also very artistic and often have a knack for writing beautiful poetry.

YOUR BEAUTY OUTLOOK: Since crabs are all about natural beauty, you like to keep your looks pretty low-key. Why not put some of that creative energy into your beauty routine? Even if you don't like to go too crazy with color, try something simple like a shimmer cream on your cheeks or go and hunt out a perfume that you really love. These are subtle ways you can express your personal style without looking over-the-top.

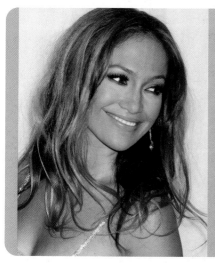

Leo ♌ JULY 24–AUGUST 23

STAR SIBLING: *Jennifer Lopez*

WHO YOU ARE: No one ever wonders where you are because you're always the center of attention. This suits you perfectly, especially since Leos love to be the leader or go-to person for whatever is going on. The good part of having all this drive is that it also makes you very giving and many Leos love to do volunteer work. The downside of being the boss type is that you love to have things go your way. Just remember to listen to other people's thoughts and opinions and you'll be class president in no time.

YOUR BEAUTY OUTLOOK: When it comes to style you are a serious glamazon. You are the first one to get a dress for every school dance and are practicing how to wear your hair weeks in advance. You will look great in dramatic eyeliner drawn across in a thin line across the top eyelid and two coats of mascara. Another trick you'll love when dressing up? Dusting the skin on your upper arms and shoulders with sparkling body powder for a little extra star power.

Virgo ♍ AUGUST 24–SEPTEMBER 23

STAR SIBLING: *Beyoncé*

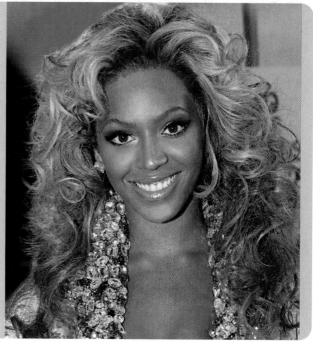

WHO YOU ARE: Those born under this sign love order. You are the type who keeps the neatest notebooks, writes down all of your homework, and never leaves sweaty gym clothes wrinkled up in your locker. Also, since you are such an intellectual whiz, you don't feel the need to follow the herd and often pick alternative paths to what everyone else is doing. However, all of that order can make you a little stressed out, so learning to chill out is a must.

YOUR BEAUTY OUTLOOK: You are the total perfectionist of the zodiac and your looks reflect that. Even when you're just showing up for class, you hair and makeup always look perfect. While you never look too funky, you're the last one who would sport smeared mascara or split ends. Since you're also quite picky, it's easy for you to spend an hour trying out testers in the drug or department store (if you have a hard time deciding, ask the woman behind the cosmetics counter for a sample). Stylewise, try something a little unexpectedly messy or colorful. Add a little pomade to the ends of your hair so they get that cool, piece-y look, or wear mascara in a subtle shade like navy or plum for an eye-opening surprise.

Libra ♎ SEPTEMBER 24–OCTOBER 23

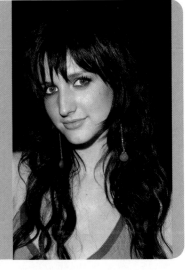

STAR SIBLING: *Ashlee Simpson*

WHO YOU ARE: In addition to being very sociable, you like your life to have balance and harmony. Since you're someone who tinkers a bit with everything (you're just as comfortable in drama class as in gym), you often have a lot of friends. With their charming personalities, Librans are also the boy-magnets of the zodiac (but not in a shallow or fake way). Libra is considered the most stylish sign, so you're always dressed for any occasion.

YOUR BEAUTY OUTLOOK: You always like to put your best face forward, so having a regular skin care routine is a good idea. Make sure to find a cleanser and moisturizer that work for you. You should also use a mild scrub or mask once a week to keep pores clear and breakout-free. You are not one to cover up under a ton of makeup, but dabbing on a little tinted moisturizer with an SPF every day will protect your face as well as cover up any minor blemishes that may pop up. Cream blush is a good idea for you since it gives a healthy glow that's next to natural. Apply a dot to the apple of your cheek and blend it in with your pointer and middle finger in a circular motion.

Scorpio ♏ OCTOBER 24–NOVEMBER 22

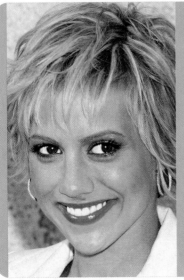

STAR SIBLING: *Brittany Murphy*

WHO YOU ARE: Scorpios are hard to typecast because you can change your personality or likes and dislikes at the drop of a hat. You like to remain a little bit of a mystery and are happy as the center of attention one minute, and then off on the sidelines the next. Your brain is always working and people often describe your personality as intense and powerful. However, underneath all that toughness is a ton of sensitivity that the rest of the world often doesn't get a chance to see.

YOUR BEAUTY OUTLOOK: You like to change your looks quite a bit but at the same time know what works for your face and your hair, so never do anything too crazy. After trying a bunch of shades and products you feel like you've finally found what works best on you. Since you're known as such a powerhouse, we suggest that you stock up on an equally bold red lipstick. The rest of your face can stay fairly naked but a bright mouth makes a great statement. The same goes for your hair—you are totally willing to change your haircolor, but not every month. Go to your stylist and ask about some highlights—these can lighten your look but don't require a ton of upkeep, since it's not your whole head that's being colored.

Sagittarius ♐ NOVEMBER 23–DECEMBER 22

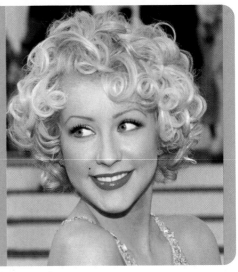

STAR SIBLING: *Christina Aguilera*

WHO YOU ARE: Sagittarius is one of the most open-minded signs of the zodiac and also the one who prefers to keep her head in the clouds instead of down on planet Earth with the rest of us (this is probably also why you are also the most optimistic sign). You have a knack for making friends and are very quick-witted. The only negative is that sometimes you blurt things out before you've really thought them through, so be careful not to hurt anyone's feelings with your spontaneous outbursts.

YOUR BEAUTY OUTLOOK: Since you're a fan of the great outdoors, remember to wear a moisturizer that also has an SPF 15 so you won't get burned. Makeup-wise, any product that multitasks is right up your alley (check out those chubby pencils that work on eyes, cheeks, and lips), but you'll also look great in pretty colored eye shadows. Light-eyed girls should try a lavender or pale blue whereas anyone with dark eyes can go for an emerald green or a gold. When it comes to hairstyles, anything that offers high impact but minimal effort is totally your style.

Capricorn ♑ DECEMBER 23–JANUARY 20

STAR SIBLING: *Kristin Kreuk*

WHO YOU ARE: You are the most logical sign of the zodiac, and like to keep all of your stuff (from homework to your wardrobe) in order. When it comes to doing a task, you're all about the details and making sure that everything is perfect. You are also the most ambitious sign of the zodiac, so are probably the one perusing all those college applications way before the rest of your friends.

YOUR BEAUTY OUTLOOK: Your love of being organized also spills into your beauty routine. You are the one who always gets regular hair trims and probably throws your mascara out every three months just like the experts suggest. Also, while goats are known for being fairly rigid when it comes to stuff like school, you also love to let your hair down and have some fun during the weekend or holidays. Next time you're visiting your stylist, ask her to show you an easy updo so you can have a party perfect 'do. When it comes to makeup, you are the perfect candidate to wear liquid eyeliner, since attention to detail will almost guarantee a perfect line.

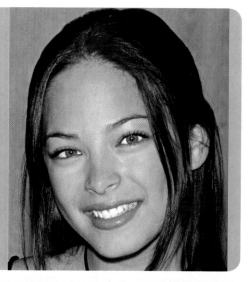

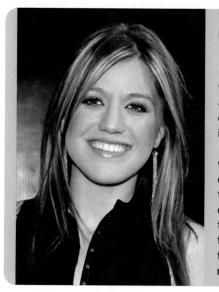

Aquarius ♒ JANUARY 21–FEBRUARY 19

STAR SIBLING: *Kelly Clarkson*

WHO YOU ARE: You're the type of girl who is always one style-step ahead of everyone else, wearing a trend before it's even a trend. Water Bearers also have a huge humanitarian streak and are often found doing volunteer work or trying to save the planet. While some may think of you as quirky, we think independent and intriguing is more to the point—and there's nothing wrong with that.

YOUR BEAUTY OUTLOOK: When it comes to your looks, you're not really concerned with what everyone else is doing. Your bathroom is filled with products but, chances are, some of them get used a couple of times and then you move onto something else. While we're totally into you trying new products, make sure to remain somewhat consistent when it comes to your skin care—it takes at least six weeks to see results from a regular skin routine, so don't change it too often. Also, since you're the type who will splurge every now and then on something amazing, check out the new custom-blended foundations that are made to match your skin tone. That way you'll have flawless skin that is just waiting for your next makeup creation.

Pisces ♓ FEBRUARY 20–MARCH 20

STAR SIBLING: *Brittany Snow*

WHO YOU ARE: Hey, fish girls! Being in this sign you are blessed with imagination, creativity, and just a touch of sophistication. You can be a bit of a dreamer but you also have a great appreciation for the arts, such as poetry, painting, or prose. You are very giving as a friend and intensely loyal—once someone has won your trust you will keep him or her in your life forever.

YOUR BEAUTY OUTLOOK: With your head in the clouds, you like to change your look depending on the day, time, and how you're feeling. Also, since Pisces girls like stuff that's on the chic side, why not hit a department store and sniff out a new scent? If you can't afford the real thing, snap up the body lotion instead. It's less expensive and will make you feel like a perfumed queen when you apply it after a shower. With your creative spirit, don't limit yourself when it comes to makeup. Try combinations like light blue eyeshadow teamed with raspberry lips. Or, a purple liner with green mascara. Trust your instincts (and great sense of color) and see what you come up with since you can make any shade combo work, thanks to your artistic mind.

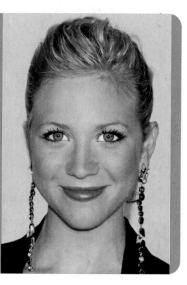

TOP 10 STYLISH FLICKS TO WATCH WITH YOUR FRIENDS

Want to make your Blockbuster night a little more beautiful? We've rounded up some of our favorite flicks that also have a serious style edge. Not only do these movies show characters with incredible flair, they also show us what was considered the height of fashion in different eras. Why is this cool? Well, with all the retro looks that keep coming back, it's fun to check out what girls really looked like back then. From the princess hairstyles of the '50s to the blue eye shadow of the '80s, all of these flicks are great examples of how styles change as well as some seriously sassy girl characters taking charge. So rent them and see if you're a Holly Golightly or an Elle Woods.

Breakfast at Tiffany's

THE STORY: This classic stars the beautiful Audrey Hepburn as Holly Golightly, making her way through a very glamorous New York City in the early '60s.

THE STYLE: All the costumes in this movie were created by Givenchy, the designer-of-the-moment back then. Simple to-the-knee cocktail dresses, cropped jackets, and amazing updos are all the rage.

COPY IT: Looking for the best prom 'do? You must see this movie. This is old-school glamour at its finest. Also, now that all the girly retro styles are coming back, this is a good way to see how the look was done originally. Think soft pink lips, and liquid eyeliner that is to die for.

Clueless

THE STORY: Alicia Silverstone plays Cher Horowitz, a Beverly Hills teen who has shopping down to a fine science. A popular girl with a heart of gold, she likes nothing better than playing matchmaker for her teachers and friends.

THE STYLE: Her closet is so enormous that her clothes hang on a revolving electric rack so she can scan hundreds of trendy outfits before deciding what to wear. This movie is all about girlie-girl style—her hair is always super straight and shiny and she wears lots of lip gloss.

COPY IT: Look pretty without piling on the makeup. Cher and her two best friends, Tai and Dionne, all sport clear skin, minimal eye makeup, and the best pouts ever.

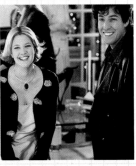

The Wedding Singer

THE STORY: In this funny flick, set in 1985, Adam Sandler and Drew Barrymore play Robbie and Julia—two people looking for love in all the wrong places, until they see each other.

THE STYLE: Drew wears tons of pastel blue eyeshadow and frosty gloss. Christine Taylor as Holly wears some of the more unfortunate styles of the '80s—hair curled to a crisp and way too much glitter.

COPY IT: Pastel eye shadows and liners are worth a try and look beyond pretty. Like Drew, keep the rest of your face fairly neutral.

Legally Blonde

THE STORY: Beverly Hills babe Elle Woods goes to Harvard to win back her boyfriend. She's a fish out of water, but while she's there, she finds her true calling and her true love.

THE STYLE: Does it get any girlier than this? High ponytails, cute suits, pink lipstick, and matching manicures are what it's all about.

COPY IT: Elle wears all the latest trends but manages to put her own stamp on everything. Follow her style rules by busting out and creating some of your own.

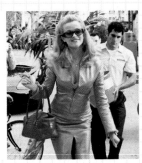

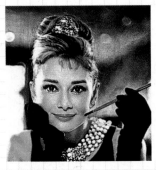

The Matrix

THE STORY: Are we living in the Matrix or not? That is the question. The space-age action, style, and, well, Keanu Reeves make this flick a must-see.

THE STYLE: Takes the term "city slicker" to a whole new level. Lots of dark clothes, preferably long coats. Makeup is kept to a neutral minimum.

COPY IT: Get the chic 'do. Apply a dollop of light-hold gel to damp hair and comb it through. Part hair on the side and slick it back. Long-haired girls can pull hair into a low ponytail, twist it, and pin it up at the base of the neck.

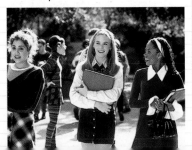

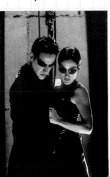

Grease

THE STORY: The goody-goody falls in love with the bad boy. Sandy and Danny (Olivia Newton-John and John Travolta) show us what high school was like 50 years ago.

THE STYLE: If you're looking for some of the coolest looks for a school dance, these vintage looks rock. The girls look so pretty in their poodle skirts and matching cardigans, while the guys look so cool in black leather and enough hair gel to put the Gotti brothers to shame.

COPY IT: If you've always wanted to try vintage style but aren't sure of where to start, this movie gives you some easy suggestions—high ponytails, shimmery cheeks, and glossy nails. Don't forget lots of pink.

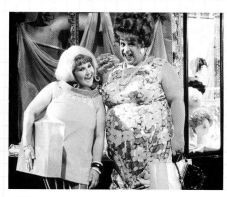

Hairspray

THE STORY: This fab movie has a pretty heavy storyline: it's all about racial segregation in the 1960s. But thanks to Tracy Turnblad (Ricki Lake), the outfits, and the twisting tunes, this movie is hilarious.

THE STYLE: It's retro all the way, with the biggest beehives, the pouffiest dresses, and over-the-top makeup looks.

COPY IT: This comedy can serve as an example of when too much of a good thing becomes a bad thing. If you are into the whole '60s vibe because it's pretty and ultra feminine (think winged-out eyeliner paired with pale pink lips), go for it.

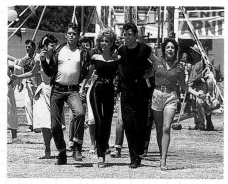

Uptown Girls

THE STORY: Brittany Murphy plays Molly Gunn, a total socialite who suddenly has no money and has to go out and get a job. She ends up as a nanny to a very grown-up girl who teaches Molly a thing or two about life.

THE STYLE: Murphy looks awesome in this. Her character puts together cool outfit combinations like embroidered denim dresses with clogs and tiny glam tanks with jeans.

COPY IT: Charlotte turns a beaded votive candleholder into a flower hairpin. We're not suggesting you start including housewares in your beauty routine, but it's a great example of how to get crafty and look totally unique.

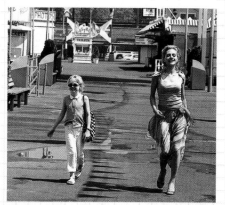

Lost in Translation

THE STORY: Our heroine, Charlotte (Scarlett Johansson), is in Tokyo while her husband works on a photo shoot. She spends her days reading fashion magazines until she bumps into fellow American Bob Harris, and they strike up an odd friendship.

THE STYLE: Charlotte is always dressed in super-simple outfits that look cute without looking like she tried (flats, pants, and a sweet sweater). It also shows us a lot of the capital of Japan, which is known as one of the hubs of street style.

COPY IT: Keep it simple. Leave your hair fairly natural—just add a tiny amount of pomade or wax to give it a messy, textured look. As for makeup, some mascara and sheer pink gloss are all you need. Stick with neutral pieces like capri pants in navy and a matching sweater with Keds.

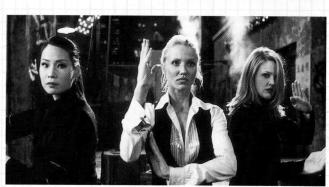

Charlie's Angels

THE STORY: Three detectives (Cameron Diaz, Drew Barrymore, and Lucy Liu) retrieve some hush-hush voice ID software. The best part is watching them kick butt and change outfits while saving the world.

THE STYLE: What style isn't represented here? There's everything from serious Disco Queen with Cameron Diaz getting down, to Drew Barrymore as a heavy-metal rocker. Since these three ladies are the masters of disguise, they get to show off a little bit of everything.

COPY IT: Whatever trend you pick from this, the main idea is to be willing to stand out in a crowd.

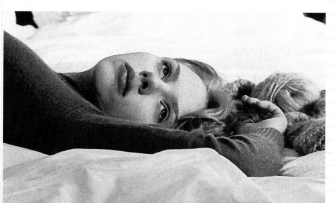

QUIZ: ARE YOU A BEAUTY CHAMELEON?

Do you change your look every time you change your socks or every time Justin Timberlake calls you up and proposes marriage (um, that means never)? While we're all for finding your style and sticking to it, there are always new tips, trends, and products to try, and we recommend a little fun experimentation every now and again. Perhaps you are the exact opposite, a regular makeup trailblazer who switches looks after watching **TRL**. Each month, **Teen People** shows the latest looks on everyone from screen sirens like Kirsten Dunst to R & B divas like Ashanti. So answer these questions and find if you're on top of the trends, how to try something new, as well as great tips that every girl needs to know.

1. HOW MANY BOTTLES OF PERFUME DO YOU OWN?
A) 8

B) 3

C) 1

2. IF YOU GOT A LAST-MINUTE DATE INVITE, WOULD YOU BE ABLE TO PULL TOGETHER A GLAM LOOK REALLY FAST?
A) I'd change out of my scruffy jeans to my nice ones

B) A quick head-to-toe makeover is no problem

C) I'd make some small but significant changes like brushing my hair and ditching my sneakers

3. HOW OFTEN DO YOU BUY NEW BEAUTY PRODUCTS?
A) Every couple of months, if I see something that's really great

B) Whenever I run out of something

C) I pick up a little something here and there

4. IF YOU COULD INVENT A BEAUTY PRODUCT, WHAT WOULD IT BE?
A) A lipstick that changes color every day (and would always look good on me)

B) Concealer that doesn't budge

C) A spray that would clean my hair without having to wash it

5. WHAT MAKEUP LOOK WOULD YOU NEVER WEAR?
A) All those dark smoky eyes look a little scary

B) Anything too bright

C) The wash 'n' go thing is not for me

YOUR SCORE: 1. A=2 B=1 C=0 2. A=0 B=2 C=1
3. A=1 B=0 C=2 4. A=2 B=1 C=0 5. A=1 B=0 C=2

Your Score . . .
0–3, Playing it safe

You still feel a little intimidated when it comes to trying all the new beauty trends that appear in magazines and on celebrities. While we totally get that not every look is for everybody, it's fun to mix it up every once in a while.

WHAT TO TRY: Something that's a subtle change. Makeup-wise, it's easy to do something small, such as change your lip gloss shade or switch from a black eyeliner to a softer brown. However, if you want to try a totally different look, check out "Your True Colors" on page 40. When it comes to your haircut, ask your stylist what small changes she could make to your hair to make a big difference in the style. Also, after your stylist is done snipping, ask her for some styling tips or what product she would recommend that you use—a little gel or pomade can add pizzazz.

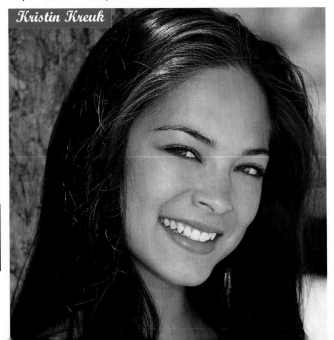

Kristin Kreuk

4–7, Willing to experiment

You are totally intrigued by hair products and makeup but often feel overwhelmed by the number of choices out there. The trick to changing without looking like you've tried too hard is to stick in your comfort zone. Go through a bunch of magazines and find a celeb who looks like you and has a similar style and coloring. See how they tweak their look for different occasions and get inspired.

WHAT TO TRY: Do you always wear mascara? Crank up your glam factor a tiny bit more by also trying a liner pencil in a dark-ish shade (gray, brown, or navy). To apply, just do small dots right at the base of the lashes—this makes them look super thick. Also, for some serious glam tips that we guarantee will look great, go to "Our All-Time Favorite Celeb Makeup Looks" on page 64.

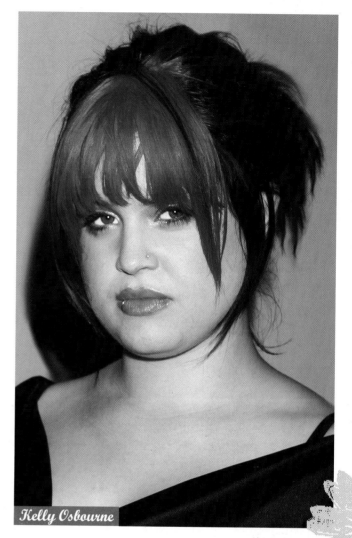

Kelly Osbourne

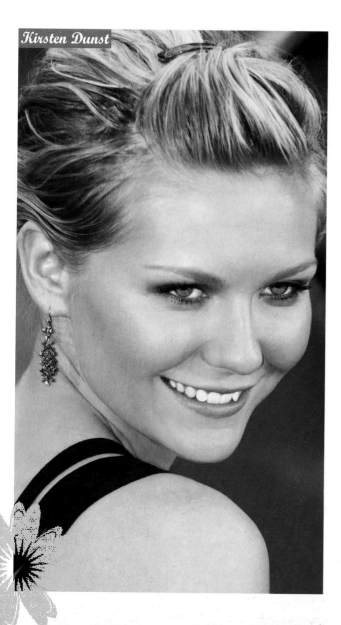

Kirsten Dunst

8–10, Total chameleon

Your mood and personality totally show through in your makeup choices and hairstyles. One minute you're sporting Gwen Stefani's red lips and the next minute you're Amy Lee from Evanescence with goth black eyeliner. If you want to really stay on top of the trends (so you can start them instead of following them), look at the latest beauty styles that are on the fashion runways. This is where the top makeup artists create the latest and greatest.

WHAT TO TRY: You need to play it safe with certain products. For example, when it comes to foundation and concealer, finding one that matches your skin perfectly can take some time. Once you've found your perfect shade, you're set. And, luckily, great skin is the perfect canvas for those hot new makeup shades. For more info on getting great looking skin, check out the "What's Your Skin Type?" quiz on page 26.

chapter seven

DO-IT-YOURSELF SPA PARTY

everything you need to plan the perfect
at-home beauty blowout

DO-IT-YOURSELF SPA PARTY

*I*nstead of having your friends over for the usual girls'-night-in of movies and popcorn, why not turn Saturday night into an evening of pampering at your very own Hollywood spa? We've made things super-easy by planning the whole evening for you–from designing the cutest invitation, to collecting ideas for delectable spa-like snacks, to making suggestions for the perfect goodie bag for your guests to take home. The spa treatments that you'll be doing come straight from spa specialists who pamper stars such as Mandy Moore, Cameron Diaz, and Hilary Duff, to name a few. Within these pages you'll find everything you need to pull off your Hollywood Spa Party without a hitch. The actual treatments have been written up in easy-to-follow recipe formats and we guarantee that you and your friends will be glowing by the time the clock strikes midnight. So, get ready to have a blast and get gorgeous!

GET READY TO FEEL LIKE A STAR!
You're invited to a Hollywood Spa Party

Date:

Time:

Place:

RSVP

PS Please remember to bring a comfy T-shirt (that you don't mind getting messy), cozy sweats, a towel, something to tie back your hair with, a favorite nail polish, and your favorite CD for relaxing.

Relax! Unwind! . . . Like the Stars!

PLANNING YOUR GUEST LIST

Think about how many of your friends you want to invite to your Hollywood Spa Party. Unlike the usual shindig, where you can have as many guests as you can cram into your living room, this pampering gathering should probably be kept on the small side. We suggest inviting three of your best friends so you'll be four girls total (yes, don't forget yourself). For one thing, you need to make enough of each recipe for all your guests, and you want to make sure to have enough room to get comfortable—to spread out all those glamorama supplies, not to mention room in the bathroom when you need it for masks. And hey, if this party goes off without a hitch, you can always throw another with a different group of girls at a later date. On the other hand, if you have the room, and you're game, you can double or triple these recipes to accommodate parties of eight or twelve.

WHAT WILL YOU BE DOING?

Your next job is to choose which treatments to do with your guests. How many will you have time for? Which ones seem right for your crowd? While we've given you a choice in each major treatment category, keep in mind that you don't need to do them all. In fact, a well-balanced combination would be to do a toner, a scrub, and a face mask. After that, your party space will determine what other treatments you include. For example, if you have a big bathroom with a tub that four of you can all sit around, it might be fun to do a spa pedicure. If you don't have the bathroom space, we give you an alternative recipe for a mini-pedicure that doesn't require major foot soaking. Or you can turn to page 128 and give each other manicures. Also, your Spa Party will be the most fun if you and your friends pair off in twos for treatments. That way, two of you are in the bathroom at the same time helping each other out. For example, leaning over the sink, you can put a gloppy mask on your friend, and she can help you with yours. The girls who are waiting can be snacking on "spa" food (there are cool recipes on pages 148–149), flipping through the latest issues of *Teen People,* or just chilling out to music. No treatment takes that long to apply, so don't expect a lot of downtime.

SPA PARTY SUPPLIES

• A stack of towels. Try to have one big and one small size for each party guest. If you are short on towels, ask your friends to bring their own.

• A box of tissues. These always come in handy for wiping up small spills, and taking off any little leftover scrub or mask bits from your face; plus they are great to use as toe separators when painting your nails.

• A box of cotton swabs. Great for dabbing on product or cleaning up your polish after you paint your nails.

• A bag of cotton balls or pads. These are the best for applying toner and removing old nail polish before a pedicure or manicure.

• A box of nail files. You need these for pedicures/manicures. With a box you can give each girl her own file to take home.

Once you've decided which treatments you want to make (recipes follow), draw up shopping lists for the items you need to buy. Everything can be found at the supermarket, health food store, drugstore or craft store. Read over the lists carefully and cross off anything that you already have on hand at home.

WONDERING WHERE TO GO TO BUY YOUR PARTY SUPPLIES?
HERE'S WHERE YOU'LL BE HEADING TO PURCHASE THE FOLLOWING ITEMS:

SUPERMARKET
❏ All fruits and vegetables
❏ Chocolate chips
❏ Oatmeal
❏ Honey
❏ Apple cider vinegar
❏ White wine vinegar
❏ Eggs
❏ Yogurt
❏ Kosher salt
❏ Olive oil
❏ Pineapple juice
❏ Maple syrup
❏ Milk

DRUGSTORE
❏ Witch hazel
❏ Vitamin E capsules
❏ Cocoa butter

HEALTH FOOD STORE
❏ Lemon essential oil
❏ Tea tree essential oil
❏ Sweet orange essential oil
❏ Dry clay
❏ Black currant herbal tea bags
❏ Fresh lavender

CRAFT STORE
❏ Small plastic pots with screw tops (like lip gloss pots)
❏ 1-oz. empty plastic bottles with screw tops
❏ Sticky labels so everyone can personalize their products
❏ Stickers, glitter, or anything else you want to use to decorate products you give your friends to take home as gifts.
❏ Dried lavender

PARTY FOOD!

Now that you've figured out what beauty treatments you are going to make, it's time to think of other things that will make your evening complete. Decide what room you are going to be using for your spa, and then it's all about making that room as comfy as possible. Place a pile of magazines in a corner (these are great for doing quizzes with each other or reading articles between treatments). Also, grab a stack of your own CDs as well as adding the ones that your friends bring along (pick tunes that are relaxing to add to the chill spa vibe). Anything that's soft to sit on like cushions and blankets (fluffy sleeping bags), can be stacked up in the corner of the room so everyone can just take their own when they arrive.

At the same time you're feeding your face with all of these good-for-you beauty treatments, you'll no doubt be getting a little hungry. We've included a few easy, spa-licious recipes below. When it comes to the snacks, feel free to add your own ideas with simple, healthy stuff like bowls of mixed nuts, trail mix, cut-up fruit, or veggies and dip. Since you probably won't be sitting down at a table, we recommend keeping your menu to finger foods that are easy to pop in your mouth.

BANANA POPS

(Makes 8 pops)

What You'll Need

- ❑ PLATES
- ❑ KNIFE
- ❑ 8 CRAFT STICKS
- ❑ SPOON
- ❑ WAXED PAPER
- ❑ BAKING SHEET

Ingredients

- ❑ 2 CUPS EACH: GROUND TOASTED ALMONDS, SHREDDED COCONUT, CANDY SPRINKLES, AND GRAHAM CRACKER CRUMBS
- ❑ 4 JUST-RIPE BANANAS, PEELED
- ❑ 1/2 CUP HONEY

To Make

1. Spread ground nuts (or other toppings of choice) on a plate or plates.

2. Cut bananas in half crosswise. Insert a craft stick into each cut end.

3. To assemble, hold each banana half over plate or waxed paper to catch drips. Spoon about 1 tablespoon honey over banana, rotating and smoothing honey with back of spoon to coat all sides. Roll banana in topping of choice until coated on all sides, pressing with fingertips to help topping adhere.

4. Place pops on waxed paper–lined baking sheet. Repeat with remaining bananas, honey, and topping.

MINI PIZZAS

(Makes 4 servings—2 mini pizzas each)

What You'll Need

- ❑ KNIFE
- ❑ SPOON
- ❑ WAXED PAPER
- ❑ BAKING SHEET

Ingredients

- ❑ 8 ENGLISH MUFFINS
- ❑ 1 JAR PIZZA SAUCE
- ❑ PEPPERONI SLICES
- ❑ CHOPPED ONIONS/GREEN PEPPERS
- ❑ OTHER DESIRED TOPPINGS
- ❑ SHREDDED MOZZARELLA
- ❑ PARMESAN CHEESE

To Make

1. Cut English muffins and toast until golden.

2. Spread desired amount of pizza sauce on each muffin half. Place on a waxed paper–lined baking sheet.

3. Top with desired toppings and sprinkle with shredded mozzarella.

4. Broil until cheese is bubbly (about 3 to 5 minutes).

5. Sprinkle on Parmesan cheese.

BERRY BLAST MILK SHAKES

(Makes 4 servings)

What You'll Need
- ❑ BLENDER
- ❑ GLASSES
- ❑ STRAWS

Ingredients
- ❑ 1 PINT NONFAT VANILLA ICE CREAM OR NONFAT FROZEN YOGURT
- ❑ 1 PINT STRAWBERRIES, HULLED; OR AN ASSORTMENT OF BERRIES, ABOUT 2½ CUPS
- ❑ ½ CUP NONFAT MILK
- ❑ ¼ CUP HONEY
- ❑ 4 SMALL MINT SPRIGS (OPTIONAL)

To Make
1. In blender, combine all ingredients except mint sprigs and blend until smooth and creamy, about 30 seconds.
2. Serve immediately in tall, chilled glasses.
3. Garnish with mint sprigs, if desired.

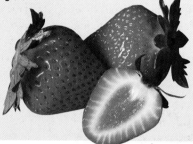

GIANT PRETZELS

(Makes 12 pretzels)

What You'll Need
- ❑ 2 MIXING BOWLS
- ❑ CLEAN DISH TOWEL
- ❑ WAXED PAPER
- ❑ BAKING SHEET

Ingredients
- ❑ 1 ENVELOPE YEAST
- ❑ 1½ CUP WARM WATER (105–115 DEGREES)
- ❑ ½ TEASPOON SUGAR (NEEDED FOR YEAST TO RISE)
- ❑ 4½ CUPS FLOUR
- ❑ 1 TBSP. OLIVE OIL
- ❑ 1 EGG YOLK
- ❑ 2 TBSP. WATER
- ❑ COARSE SALT AND SESAME SEEDS

To Make
1. In one of the bowls, dissolve yeast in warm water and add sugar. Add flour and knead 6 minutes.
3. Grease clean bowl with olive oil. Place dough in bowl., cover with a dish towel and let rise until doubled in size.
4. Divide the dough into 12 pieces and roll them into long sticks. Arrange pretzels on the waxed paper–lined baking sheet as sticks or twist them to look like traditional pretzels.
5. Beat together the egg and the water with a fork and brush some of the mixture onto the pretzels. Sprinkle each pretzel with coarse salt or sesame seeds.
6. Bake at 450°F for 12 minutes. Note: You can heat these up again when your friends arrive.

CRUNCHY POPCORN BALLS

(Makes 20 balls)

What You'll Need
- ❑ SAUCEPAN
- ❑ MIXING BOWL
- ❑ WOODEN MIXING SPOON
- ❑ WAXED PAPER
- ❑ BAKING SHEET

Ingredients
- ❑ 5 QUARTS POPPED POPCORN
- ❑ ¾ CUP LIGHT CORN SYRUP
- ❑ ¼ CUP MARGARINE, PLUS MORE FOR YOUR HANDS
- ❑ 2 TSP. COLD WATER
- ❑ 2½ CUPS CONFECTIONERS' SUGAR
- ❑ 1 CUP MARSHMALLOWS

To Make
1. In a saucepan over medium heat, combine the corn syrup, margarine, cold water, confectioners' sugar, and marshmallows. Stir just until the mixture comes to a boil. Remove from heat.
2. In mixing bowl, carefully combine the hot mixture with the popcorn, coating each kernel.
3. Using a spoon, scoop out small amounts onto a waxed paper–lined baking sheet and allow them to cool.
4. Smear your hands with margarine and shape into 20 balls.

YOUR AT-HOME SPA TIMETABLE

BELOW IS A TIMELINE OF WHAT YOUR EVENING COULD LOOK LIKE. THIS WAY YOU'LL BE TOTALLY ORGANIZED BUT STILL ABLE TO HAVE A BLAST. "IT'S A GOOD IDEA TO MAKE A LOT OF THE PRODUCTS AHEAD OF TIME," SAYS SONYA DAKAR, WHO IS DREW BARRYMORE AND ELISHA CUTHBERT'S FACIALIST. "THAT WAY THE EVENING WILL RUN SMOOTHLY AND THERE WON'T BE A HUGE MESS TO CLEAN UP AT THE END."

NOON TO 4 PM

Time to start whipping up all the snacks that you want to serve your friends. Make all of the food that is supposed to be served cold first so that way it has time to cool down in the refrigerator. Anything that needs to be served warm can just be placed on the kitchen counter (cover it in tinfoil when you are done cooking) or in the oven with the power off. If you're going to have snacks like chips or nuts, put them in bowls now and set them out in the room where all of you guys are going to be doing your spa stuff, so it will be done. Also, assemble anything that you want to put in each girl's goody bag.

4 PM TO 5 PM

Mix up most of your at-home beauty products. We suggest that you create at least a toner, a scrub, and a mask. For example, a beautiful evening could include:

- ❏ Tropical Toner
- ❏ Honey and Oatmeal Scrub
- ❏ Avocado and Egg Facial Mask

Once you've whipped up these three recipes, place them all in airtight containers and store them in the refrigerator. If you want to make more treats why not add some of the other recipes:

- ❏ Fab Foot Fixer
- ❏ Chocolate Lip Balm
- ❏ All-Natural Zit Zapper

5 PM TO 6 PM

Now is the time to set up the room where you and your friends are going to be with everything we listed before (towels, CDs, etc). Also, do a bathroom check to make sure tissues, cotton balls, and any other necessary tools are easily accessible.

6 PM TO 7 PM

Put the food out. Make sure to provide lots of plates, forks, and napkins. Set up glasses in the kitchen so it's easy for your friends to get their drinks.

7 PM TO 8 PM

Everyone is here! While you and your friends are catching up and chatting, bring the beauty treatments out and set them up on a table. Don't forget to turn on the CD player with someone's favorite songs!

8 PM TO 8:30 PM

Every girl should wash her face, grab a cotton ball, and swipe her face with toner. Next, go into the bathroom in pairs and try out the scrub.

8:30 PM TO 9 PM

Time to apply a mask. This is also a perfect time to pop in a DVD and start your movie, since you have to sit still while the mask dries and does its thing. For ideas on what movies to rent, check out "Top 10 Stylish Flicks To Watch With Your Friends" on page 140.

9 PM TO 9:30 PM

If you made the Fab Foot Fixer, now is the time to get it out. Set up a bowl of the scrub and the sliced-up lemons in your bathroom. If there's a bathtub handy, chances are three or four of you can go at the same time. If you are skipping this recipe, go onto the Mini Pedi.

9:30 PM TO 10 PM

Time to get crafty and decorate your lip gloss pots before you start cooking. Use whatever you want, such as markers, stickers or glitter, felt shapes, and glue. When everyone is finished, go to the kitchen and mix up the Chocolate Lip Balm (see page 157).

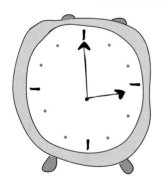

10 PM AND ON

If some of your friends are going home, give them a goody bag of samples to take with them. If some are sleeping over, don't forget to dab on a tiny bit of the All-Natural Zit Zapper before you hit the sheets. That way you'll all wake up and be truly gorgeous!

BEAUTY RECIPES

WHEN COLLECTING RECIPES THAT WERE STARWORTHY, WE WENT STRAIGHT TO THE TOP SOURCES. BRIGITTE BEASSE OF THE ONA SPA/PRIVE SALON, ONE OF THE COOLEST HOLLYWOOD BEAUTY SPOTS, WHERE HILARY DUFF, TARA REID, LUCY LIU AND MANDY MOORE HAVE ALL BEEN SEEN, GAVE US A FEW GREAT IDEAS. "IT'S SO MUCH FUN TO MAKE A SPA IN YOUR HOME," SAYS BEASSE. "NOT ONLY DO YOU AND YOUR FRIENDS GET A CHANCE TO REALLY BOND, BUT YOU'RE ALSO DOING SOMETHING GREAT FOR YOUR SKIN." JULIE SERQUINA OF THE PAINT SHOP BEVERLY HILLS, WHERE CAMERON DIAZ GETS HER PIGGIES POLISHED, ALSO HOOKED US UP WITH SOME MORE DO-IT-YOURSELF SUPERSTAR TREATMENTS. FOLLOW THE RECIPES BELOW AND YOU'LL BE FEELING PAMPERED IN NO TIME. EACH RECIPE MAKES ENOUGH FOR FOUR PEOPLE.

IRRITATION ALERT!

Before you start smearing on these delicious beauty treats, ask your friends if they are allergic to any of the ingredients. If you are unsure, it's a good idea to do an allergy spot test. To do this, just apply a small amount of the mixture on the inside of your lower arm. Let it sit there for half an hour and if there's no reaction, feel free to apply the product elsewhere. If at any point during your spa night one of you feels a burning sensation from any of the treatments, rinse off immediately with cool water.

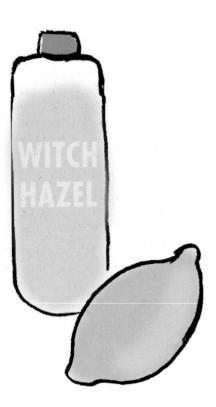

Lemon Toner

(Makes 4 1-oz. bottles)
Good For: Oily and combination skin types

This is great to use after you have washed your face (morning and night). The witch hazel acts as an astringent to clean off any dirt from your face that your cleanser may have missed. Also, lemon oil is antibacterial, so it will help to keep breakouts at bay. This is perfect for any sporty girl to keep in her gym bag to swipe her face with after a workout. The recipe makes four bottles of toner, so you and your friends can use some during the party and then everyone gets to take her bottle home, too. If you make it ahead of time, feel free to put it in the refrigerator to make it feel super cool when you put it on, but it's also OK stored on the bathroom shelf.

What You'll Need
❑ 4 1-OZ. PLASTIC BOTTLES WITH FLIP OR TWIST TOPS

Ingredients
❑ 4 OZ. WITCH HAZEL
❑ 12 DROPS LEMON ESSENTIAL OIL

To Mix
1. Pour 1 oz. of witch hazel into each bottle.
2. Add 3 drops lemon essential oil into each bottle and shake well.

To Use
Soak a cotton ball with the Lemon Toner. On a clean face, swipe the cotton ball on forehead, cheeks, nose, and chin. You may do this more than once if skin still feels greasy.

How Long It Lasts
Since there are no fresh ingredients in this mixture, this toner will last a week.

Honey and Oatmeal Scrub

(Makes 4 "servings")

Good For: All skin types except those with severe acne. Great for blackheads.

Using a mild scrub like this one helps to buff off any dead skin flakes, which can get stuck in pores and lead to acne. Oatmeal is a really gentle way to scrub and honey is both antiseptic and moisturizing. Note: Anyone who has severe acne with whiteheads should not use scrubs. The action of exfoliating can scrape off the top of a pimple, exposing the bacteria to the rest of your face. Instead, skip scrubs and try a mask instead.

What You'll Need
- ❏ MEASURING CUP
- ❏ MIXING BOWL
- ❏ WOODEN MIXING SPOON
- ❏ PLASTIC CONTAINER FOR STORING SCRUB

Ingredients
- ❏ 6 TBSP. PLAIN, PLAIN OLD-FASHIONED OATMEAL (NOT INSTANT)
- ❏ 2 TBSP. HONEY
- ❏ ½ CUP WARM WATER
- ❏ 2 TSP. WHITE WINE VINEGAR
- ❏ 2 TBSP. FRESH-SQUEEZED LEMON JUICE

To Mix
Combine all the ingredients in a bowl and stir with the spoon until it forms a thick paste.

To Use
Scoop out a handful of scrub and rub hands together to distribute it evenly onto both palms. On a clean face, spread the scrub over your entire face, covering all areas (but avoiding the delicate area around your eyes). Gently massage scrub into the skin using a circular motion. Pay particular attention to the areas where you are most prone to blackheads. Do this for about a minute before rinsing your face with warm water. Pat your face dry with a towel.

How Long It Lasts
Lemon juice helps to preserve the scrub a little bit longer, so it can sit in the fridge for three days.

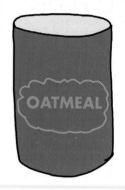

Tropical Toner

(Makes 4 1-oz. bottles)

Good For: Acne-prone, oily, or combination skin

This is another toner that is great for oily skin. Pineapple has antiseptic qualities so it helps to kill bacteria that cause acne. This tropical fruit also contains vitamins A, B, and C, which all help to protect and heal the skin (good if you picked a zit). Black currant tea is very astringent, so it helps to tighten the pores. Refrigerate when you're done making this, because it feels extra-special going on your face if it's a bit chilled. It's OK for it to sit on a shelf otherwise.

What You'll Need
- ❏ SAUCEPAN OR KETTLE
- ❏ MEASURING CUP
- ❏ MIXING BOWL
- ❏ 4 1-OZ. PLASTIC BOTTLES WITH FLIP OR TWIST TOPS
- ❏ FUNNEL

Ingredients
- ❏ 2 CUPS PURE PINEAPPLE JUICE (NOT FROM CONCENTRATE)
- ❏ 2 BLACK CURRANT HERBAL TEA BAGS

To Mix
Boil water in saucepan or kettle. Place black currant tea bags in measuring and pour 2 cups boiling water over them. Let the tea bags steep in the water for 10 minutes. Remove the tea bags and let the tea stand for another 10 minutes to cool completely. Pour the tea into a mixing bowl. Add the pineapple juice and stir to mix. Refrigerate the mixture until cooled. Divide the cooled mixture among the plastic bottles. (Use the measuring cup and a funnel to make pouring easier.)

To Use
Soak a cotton ball with the Tropical Toner. On a clean face, swipe the cotton ball on forehead, cheeks, nose, and chin. You may do this more than once if skin still feels greasy. Rinse with warm water when you're done and pat dry with a towel.

How Long It Lasts
Since it contains pure fruit juice, store this in the fridge for two days max.

MAPLE OAT FACIAL SCRUB

(Makes 4 "servings")
Good For: All skin types except those with severe acne. Great for blackheads.

Just like honey, maple syrup is great for cleansing the skin while the oatmeal gently scrubs off any dead skin flakes. The citrus essential oils keep bacteria and breakouts at bay. Note: Anyone who has severe acne with whiteheads should not use scrubs. The action of exfoliating can scrape off the top of a pimple, exposing the bacteria to the rest of your face. Instead, skip scrubs and try a mask instead.

What You'll Need
❏ MICROWAVE-SAFE BOWL
❏ WOODEN MIXING SPOON
❏ PLASTIC STORAGE CONTAINER WITH LID

Ingredients
❏ 2 TBSP. MILK
❏ 2 TBSP. PURE MAPLE SYRUP
❏ 6 TBSP. PLAIN OLD-FASHIONED NATURAL OATMEAL (NOT INSTANT)
❏ 4 DROPS LEMON ESSENTIAL OIL
❏ 2 DROPS SWEET ORANGE ESSENTIAL OIL

To Mix
In a microwave-safe bowl, warm the milk for about 20 seconds. (Do not burn or boil it.) Add the maple syrup to the milk and stir until syrup is dissolved. Add oatmeal and stir. Let sit for 5 minutes. Add essential oils and stir again to mix thoroughly.

To Use
Scoop out a handful of scrub and rub hands together to distribute it evenly onto both palms. On a clean face, spread the scrub over your entire face, covering all areas (but avoiding the delicate area around your eyes). Gently massage scrub into the skin using a circular motion. Pay particular attention to the areas where you are most prone to blackheads. Do this for about a minute before rinsing face with warm water and pat your face dry with a towel.

How Long It Lasts
Since this scrub has milk in it, we suggest ditching it when you're done, because it can sour quickly.

AVOCADO AND EGG FACIAL MASK

(Makes 4 "servings")
Good For: Oily and combination skin

This mask is great for oily or acne-prone skin. The clay in this recipe helps to absorb excess surface oil on the skin, while the avocado and egg yolk add great natural moisturizers (that aren't greasy) via vitamin E. However, if you have super dry skin it may not be the right choice. Try the Honey Yogurt Facial Mask instead.

What You'll Need
❏ MIXING BOWL
❏ WHISK
❏ WOODEN MIXING SPOON
❏ PLASTIC CONTAINER WITH A LID FOR STORING

Ingredients
❏ 3 TBSP. DRY CLAY
❏ 3 EGG YOLKS
❏ 1 SMALL AVOCADO, PITTED, PEELED, AND MASHED WITH A FORK
❏ 1 CUP WITCH HAZEL

To Mix
In the bowl, whisk together the clay and egg yolks until totally blended. Stir in the mashed avocado and slowly add the witch hazel, stirring until it forms a smooth mixture. Place in container. (Use the mask within a few hours).

To Use
On a clean face, apply a thin to medium layer of the mask all over the face with your hands, except for directly around the eye area. Let the mask sit on the face for 5 to 10 minutes and then rinse off with warm water. Gently pat face dry with a towel. If your face feels really dry, you can apply a light moisturizer.

How Long It Lasts
With all these fresh-from-the-fridge ingredients, throw any extra mask away after using.

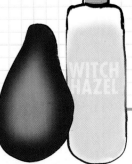

HONEY YOGURT FACIAL MASK

(Makes 4 "servings")
Good For: Normal or combination skin

Yogurt contains tons of antibacterial agents that help to zap any germs that are on the skin. Honey is also a natural moisturizer, but it's not greasy, so it won't make you break out. Lavender is great to reduce any skin inflammation or redness that is caused by acne.

Stuff You'll Need

❏ MEASURING CUP
❏ MIXING BOWL
❏ WOODEN MIXING SPOON
❏ SHARP KNIFE
❏ FORK FOR MASHING
❏ PLASTIC CONTAINER WITH A LID FOR STORING

Ingredients

❏ 4 TSP. FINELY MINCED FRESH LAVENDER BLOSSOMS (YOU CAN CHOP THEM USING A SHARP KNIFE.) IF YOU CAN'T FIND FRESH LAVENDER, THE DRIED VARIETY WILL DO.
❏ 1 CUP PLAIN YOGURT
❏ ½ CUP MASHED FRESH APRICOTS, PEACHES, OR BANANAS
❏ ½ CUP HONEY

To Mix

In a mixing bowl, combine the lavender and the yogurt and let it sit on the kitchen counter for 1 hour. Stir in the mashed-up fruit of your choice until well blended. Pour in the honey and stir again.

To Use

On a freshly washed face, patted dry but slightly damp, apply a thin layer of the mixture all over your face (avoiding the area directly around your eyes). Let the mask sit for 15–20 minutes before rinsing off with warm water. If skin feels dry, apply a light moisturizer.

How Long It Lasts

Since this scrub contains yogurt, we suggest ditching it when you're done, because it can sour quickly.

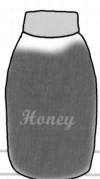

MINI PEDI

Good For: Everyone

The beauty of this foot-favoring treatment is that it doesn't need to be done in the bathroom—it's actually a good one to end your evening with, since you can do it all together while sitting around and chatting or watching a DVD.

What You'll Need

❏ BODY LOTION OR FOOT CREAM
❏ COTTON BALLS
❏ NAIL POLISH REMOVER
❏ FACIAL TISSUE
❏ NAIL FILE
❏ NAIL POLISH

To Use

Soak a cotton ball in nail polish remover and remove any existing nail polish from your toenails. File nails into desired shape if necessary. Next, put some lotion into the palm of your hand and massage it into your feet (it's also fun for you to do this to a friend's feet while she does it to yours). When finished, take another cotton ball, soak it with nail polish remover, and wipe it over toenails to get rid of the lotion (the oil will keep the polish from sticking). To separate your toes a little bit and makes it easier to apply nail polish, take a tissue and twist it up so it looks like a straw and loop it over and under your toes, starting with the big toe and working over to your little one. Start painting!

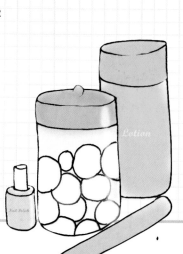

ALL-NATURAL ZIT ZAPPER

(Makes 4 1-oz. bottles)
Good For: Anyone with pesky breakouts

This is super-easy to make and is an all-natural alternative to a regular zit cream. Both ingredients are not only antibacterial, they both work to dry out areas as well. This recipe is a good one to make ahead of time and then give to all your guests to take home in their goody bags.

What You'll Need

❏ 4 1-OZ. PLASTIC BOTTLES
❏ SMALL FUNNEL
❏ COTTON SWABS

Ingredients

❏ 4 OZ. APPLE CIDER VINEGAR
❏ 40 DROPS TEA TREE ESSENTIAL OIL

To Mix

Pour 2 tablespoons (1 ounce) of cider vinegar into each bottle. Add 10 drops of tea tree oil. Close bottle and shake to mix.

To Use

Dip a cotton swab into the Zit Zapper mixture and then dab it on your blemish. Leave it on overnight and when you wake up your blemish should be much less noticeable—perhaps even gone!

How Long It Lasts

This mixture can last a week sitting in your bathroom.

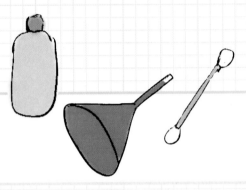

FAB FOOT FIXER

(makes 4 "servings")
Good For: everyone (space permitting)

The salt and oil mixture works to scrub off all those hard bits of skin on heels and the bottom of your feet; plus, it's moisturizing. The limes help to break down snagged cuticle skin. This foot treatment is great to do with all of your friends (or two at a time) sitting around the edge of the bathtub (if your bathroom is cramped, try the Mini Pedicure on page 155). When you're done with the Fab Foot Fixer, paint your nails (see page 129 for the ultimate set of instructions).

What You'll Need

❏ MIXING BOWL
❏ WOODEN MIXING SPOON
❏ SHARP KNIFE
❏ SMALL BOWL
❏ PLASTIC CONTAINER WITH A LID FOR STORING

Ingredients

❏ 2 CUPS KOSHER SALT
❏ 2 CUPS OLIVE OIL
❏ 3 LIMES

To Mix

In a mixing bowl, combine the salt and oil. Mix until well blended. Cut the limes into quarters and put aside in a small bowl.

To Use

Soak feet in warm water for 5 to 10 minutes to soften up the skin (it's easiest to just fill up the bathtub a couple of inches). Drain the bath and grab the limes. Take a wedge of lime and rub it over the nails and cuticles (use as many slices as you feel you need). Now take a scoop of the scrub in your hands and rub it on both feet. Massage the scrub all over your feet, especially on rough spots like heels and the balls of your feet. After a minute or two, rinse feet with cool water. Take a towel and dry your feet thoroughly.

How Long It Lasts

This foot scrub can be kept in an airtight container in your bathroom for two days max.

CHOCOLATE LIP BALM

(Makes 4 lip glosses)
Good For: everyone

This lip lube not only tastes fantastic, the vitamin E oil is great for soothing dry, chapped lips. Also, this is the perfect gift for all of your girlfriends to take home at the end of the spa, so get creative with the containers you put the gloss in. Note: If you want to do any cooking at your party, this is a great one to make with your friends around. If you are crunched for time, however, make it beforehand and stash it in their goody bags.

Stuff You'll Need

- ❏ SMALL SAUCEPAN
- ❏ WOODEN MIXING SPOON
- ❏ SMALL SPOON
- ❏ 4 SMALL PLASTIC POTS WITH SCREW TOPS (AT A CRAFT STORE)

Ingredients

- ❏ 12 TBSP. COCOA BUTTER
- ❏ 20 CHOCOLATE CHIPS
- ❏ 4 VITAMIN E CAPSULES

To Mix

Put all the ingredients in a saucepan. Turn the stove to low heat and stir with a wooden spoon until ingredients are melted and combined. Spoon into plastic pots and refrigerate until solid.

To Use

Smear on your lips whenever they feel dry or you need a chocolate fix.

How Long It Lasts

Use it every day and it will last about a month, which is perfect. Remember, it will melt if kept in a hot car or left in the sun.

THE LEFTOVERS

Just as you wouldn't eat week-old pizza that's been sitting in the fridge, the same goes for these beauty treatments. Since most of them contain food ingredients, you have to think of them the same way as food. They will spoil. Most of them are only good for one to two days after they are made, so be prepared to use them or lose them—if you don't finish them up, toss them in the trash. Anyway, now that you've made them once and know how easy it is to be a kitchen beauty queen, you won't mind whipping them up on a regular basis.

The Goodbye Gift

Give your friends a spa-themed goody bag when they leave your house. Fill it with a nail file as well as some of the recipes you made in the small plastic bottles (such as the toners and the Zit Zapper). Also, why not write up some of the other recipes on cute note cards and put them in the bags so your friends can make treatments at home? Other suggestions: Include a mini nail polish, some beauty-inspired candy (chocolate kisses and wax lips), or travel-sized products from the drugstore (body lotion, hand cream, or a purse-size brush). Also, lots of department store beauty brands have small samples that they willingly give away, so you can always hit the mall ahead of time and stockpile a few.

What should your goody bag look like? Get creative! An easy idea is to take a brown paper lunch bag, stuff it with bright colored tissue paper and then write the name of your friend on the front of the bag. Or pick up something neat at the craft store. White cardboard Chinese food containers make super-cool goody boxes.

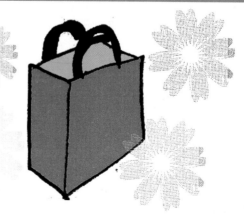

ʏTimeInc. HOME ENTERTAINMENT

TIME INC HOME ENTERTAINMENT
Publisher: Richard Fraiman
Executive Director, Marketing Services: Carol Pittard
Director, Retail & Special Sales: Tom Mifsud
Marketing Director, Branded Businesses: Swati Rao
Assistant Financial Director: Steven Sandonato
Prepress Manager: Emily Rabin
Product Manager: Victoria Alfonso
Associate Book Production Manager: Suzanne Janso
Associate Prepress Manager: Anne-Michelle Gallero
Assistant Marketing Manager: Alexandra Bliss

Special thanks: Bozena Bannett, Glenn Buonocore, Bernadette Corbie, Peter Harper, Robert Marasco, Brooke McGuire, Jonathan Polsky

Copyright 2005
Time Inc. Home Entertainment

Published by Teen People Books
Teen People Books is a trademark of Time Inc.
Time Inc.
1271 Avenue of the Americas
New York, New York 10020

ISBN: 1-932273-39-5

We welcome your comments and suggestions about Teen People Books.
Please write to us at:
Teen People Books
Attention: Book Editors
PO Box 11016
Des Moines, IA 50336-1016

FOR TEEN PEOPLE
Managing Editor: Amy Barnett
Creative Director: Jill Armus
Executive Editor: Angela Burt-Murray
Deputy Editor: Nina Malkin
Beauty Director: Tia Williams Cabezas
Photography Director: Doris Brautigan

FOR ROUNDTABLE PRESS, INC.
Directors: Julie Merberg, Marsha Melnick
Executive Editor: Patty Brown
Editor: Sara Newberry
Design: Platinum Design, Inc. NYC
Art Director: Arya Vilay
Text: Lauren McCann and Maria Neuman
Product photography: Anthony Verdez
Food photography: FoodPix
Illustrations: Arya Vilay

PHOTO CREDITS